Active Living, Cognitive Functioning, and Aging

Aging, Exercise, and Cognition Series

VOLUME 1

Leonard W. Poon, PhD

Waneen W. Spirduso, EdD

Wojtek Chodzko-Zajko, PhD

SERIES EDITORS

Active Living, Cognitive Functioning, and Aging

Leonard W. Poon, PhD
University of Georgia

Wojtek Chodzko-Zajko, PhD
University of Illinois at Urbana-Champaign

Phillip D. Tomporowski, PhD
University of Georgia

EDITORS

**HUMAN
KINETICS**

BP45

Library of Congress Cataloging-in-Publication Data

Active living, cognitive functioning, and aging / [edited by] Leonard W. Poon, Wojtek Chodzko-Zajko, Phillip D. Tomporowski

   p. ; cm. -- (Aging, exercise, and cognition ; v. 1)

   Includes bibliographical references and index.

   ISBN 0-7360-5785-4 (hard cover)

   1. Aging--Physiological aspects. 2. Aging--Psychological aspects. 3. Exercise--Physiological aspects. 4. Exercise--Psychological aspects. 5. Cognition in old age.

   [DNLM: 1. Aging--physiology. 2. Cognition--physiology. 3. Exercise--physiology. 4. Health Behavior. 5. Neurobiooogy--methods. 6. Physical Fitness. WT 104 A1895 2006] I. Poon, Leonard W., 1942- II. Chodzko-Zajko, Wojtek J. III. Tomporowski, Phillip D., 1948 IV. Series.

   QP86.A26 2006

   612.6'7--dc22

2005016219

ISBN-10: 0-7360-5785-4
ISBN-13: 978-0-7360-5785-1

Copyright © 2006 by Leonard W. Poon, Wojtek Chodzko-Zajko, and Phillip D. Tomporowski

The Web addresses cited in this text were current as of October 28, 2005, unless otherwise noted.

Acquisitions Editor: Judy Patterson Wright, PhD; **Managing Editor:** Amanda S. Ewing; **Copyeditor:** Annette Pierce; **Proofreader:** Sarah Wiseman; **Indexer:** Robert Howerton; **Permission Manager:** Dalene Reeder; **Graphic Designer:** Nancy Rasmus; **Graphic Artist:** Kathleen Boudreau-Fuoss; **Photo Manager:** Sarah Ritz; **Cover Designer:** Robert Reuther; **Art Manager:** Kelly Hendren; **Illustrator:** Al Wilborn; **Printer:** Versa Press

Printed in the United States of America   10 9 8 7 6 5 4 3 2 1

Human Kinetics

Web site: www.HumanKinetics.com

United States: Human Kinetics, P.O. Box 5076, Champaign, IL 61825-5076
800-747-4457
e-mail: humank@hkusa.com

Canada: Human Kinetics
475 Devonshire Road Unit 100, Windsor, ON N8Y 2L5
800-465-7301 (in Canada only)
e-mail: orders@hkcanada.com

Europe: Human Kinetics
107 Bradford Road, Stanningley, Leeds LS28 6AT, United Kingdom
+44 (0) 113 255 5665
e-mail: hk@hkeurope.com

Australia: Human Kinetics
57A Price Avenue, Lower Mitcham, South Australia 5062
08 8277 1555
e-mail: liaw@hkaustralia.com

New Zealand: Human Kinetics
Division of Sports Distributors NZ Ltd., P.O. Box 300 226 Albany, North Shore City, Auckland
0064 9 448 1207
e-mail: info@humankinetics.co.nz

5/19/11

CONTENTS

Contents

FOREWORD

Simply put, the topics chosen and discussed in *Active Living, Cognitive Functioning, and Aging* could not be of greater importance. The basic and applied science, which is inherent in this exploding field, is compelling. But of even greater significance are the immense social and economic implications that these topics convey. Whether our emerging billions of older selves will constitute a resource or a burden to global society is directly dependent on the issues provocatively discussed in this and subsequent volumes. To reiterate, nothing could be of greater importance to the imperatives imposed by global aging than the issues discussed in this work.

Since the early demonstrations of Diamond and others, the adaptability of the brain has been affirmed. No longer is the brain perceived to be an unknowable, passive, black-box switching center, but it is revealed as a dynamic processing organ of incredible reactive capacity. The entire domain of phenotypic plasticity asserts the intimate host-environment interface. The organism and all its constituent parts reflect what it does. The brain, no less than a muscle or an artery, mirrors the interreactivity with its constantly changing environment. Both structurally and functionally, the central nervous system obeys the "use it or lose it" dictum. Environmental enrichment sprouts new dendrites. Deprivation stumps them. And a prime aspect of such environmental enrichment is the demands imposed by movement, which as we know can increase total body energy expenditure by twentyfold over a short interval and by sixfold for the entire two-week duration of the Tour de France cycling race. The brain shares, and in many ways shapes, this energetic translation.

Numerous neuroimaging studies demonstrate the anatomical and physiological responses to movement. Fiddlers have an expanded amount of cortical tissue dedicated to the field representing the left hand. Growth factor levels, neurotransmitter metabolism, cerebral blood flow, and substrate utilization all are shown to be direct adaptive reactions to physical activity. A brain builds itself in accordance with energetic stimulation.

A hypothesis I find attractive is that the species-identifying large size of the human brain may be an evolutionary response to the exercise habits of our *Homo erectus* ancestors on the Serengeti savanna. Importantly, predatory animals have larger brains than prey. Domestication similarly leads to decreased brain size. The size of primate brains relates to the dimensions of their food-finding range of movement. These and a cascade of new reports linking physical activity to all aspects of cognitive competence come at a propitious moment. The aging of the population is linked to the surge in the incidence of the neurodegenerative diseases, which impose huge personal and national burdens. There are early reports in the scientific literature of the benefits an active lifestyle provides to persons with Alzheimer's disease and Parkinson's disease and even suggestions that physical activity may help to prevent their occurrence. The details of these possible connections are to be worked out, but the importance of the entire topic cannot possibly be overstated.

This volume and its successors inform us on these vital issues. The editors and contributors are among the world's leading experts in the area. Their papers provide a coherent glimpse into the vast vistas that remain to be explored. This work provides not only a view into who and why we are, but more excitingly, into who we may yet become.

Walter M. Bortz, II, MD
Stanford University
School of Medicine
Palo Alto, California

CONTRIBUTORS

Yagesh Bhambhani, PhD
Professor of Occupational Therapy
University of Alberta
Alberta, Canada

Wojtek J. Chodzko-Zajko, PhD
Professor and Head of Kinesiology
University of Illinois
Urbana, Illinois

M. Elaine Cress, PhD
Associate Professor of Kinesiology
Faculty of Gerontology
The University of Georgia
Athens, Georgia

Rod K. Dishman, PhD
Professor of Exercise Science
The University of Georgia
Athens, Georgia

Robert E. Dustman, PhD
Professor Emeritus in Neurology
and Research Professor in Exercise
and Sport Science
University of Utah
Salt Lake City, Utah

Carol Ann Harrington, MS
Research Associate in Gerontology
The University of Georgia
Athens, Georgia

Philip V. Holmes, PhD
Associate Professor of Psychology
The University of Georgia
Athens, Georgia

Kevin McCully, PhD
Professor of Kinesiology
The University of Georgia
Athens, Georgia

L. Stephen Miller, PhD
Associate Professor of Psychology
Faculty of Gerontology
The University of Georgia
Athens, Georgia

Patrick J. O'Conner, PhD
Professor of Kinesiology
The University of Georgia
Athens, Georgia

Leonard W. Poon, PhD
Professor of Public Health and
Psychology
Chair, Faculty of Gerontology
Director, Institute of Gerontology
The University of Georgia
Athens, Georgia

Waneen W. Spirduso, EdD
Regents Professor for Education
Research
Department of Kinesiology and
Health Science
The University of Texas
Austin, Texas

Phillip D. Tomporowski, PhD
Associate Professor of Kinesiology
Faculty of Gerontology
The University of Georgia
Athens, Georgia

Andrea White, PhD
Research Assistant Professor
of Exercise and Sports Science
University of Utah
Salt Lake City, Utah

PREFACE

Robert Butler, the first director of the National Institute on Aging, asked, "Why survive?" in his 1975 Pulitzer-winning book of the same title. Answers to *why* are intimately related to knowing *how*. Many would respond that successful survival until old age requires a healthy body and mind in order to maintain a satisfactory quality of life. Although many factors contribute to the maintenance of healthy body and mind in old age, an active lifestyle has been suggested as one of the main contributing factors.

Just how does an active lifestyle contribute to and sustain cognitive functions in old age? Although this question is quite simple, the answers are not exactly clear nor simple. This volume is the first of three that are planned to address our current knowledge of and new directions in the relationships among exercise, fitness, and cognition among older adults. Our collaborators in the planning of this series include Waneen W. Spirduso (volume II) and Arthur Kramer (volume III). The impetus for our series is that the field is ripe for breakthrough research to identify mechanisms of fitness on cognition among older adults. These breakthroughs should have an immense impact on the public health of older adults.

To systematically identify key issues, this first volume is devoted to reviews of cognitive, neurobiological, and measurement issues. The second volume is devoted to the influences of fitness on physical and mental resources as well as disease states, which in turn could affect cognitive processes. This volume focuses on direct and indirect effects of exercise and fitness as well as influences of individual differences. Finally, volume III concludes the series by examining methods to enhance cognitive and brain plasticity in older adults. Taken together, we hope to provide a series that will provide background information and different ways to pose research questions and will enhance creativity in advancing our knowledge in this field.

Chapters in volume I are divided into three parts. Chapters 1 to 3 focuses on cognitive mechanisms of the exercise–cognition relationships. Chapter 1 (Chodzko-Zajko) begins with a summary of the impact of exercise and activity on the health and well-being of older adults. There is a substantial body of scientific evidence that demonstrates the beneficial impact of regular physical activities that can bring dramatic health benefits. Despite these well-known health benefits, there has been little success in convincing older adults to adopt physically active lifestyles. Chapter 1 summarizes a *National Blueprint* that outlines the known health benefits, barriers to participation in physical activities by older adults, and strategies to increase physical activity levels. Important for this volume, chapter 1 introduces and identifies key issues relating physical activities and cognitive functioning among older adults—a set of issues not well known among the lay public and in need of both basic and applied research. The key issues identified in chapter 1 are explored in detail in subsequent chapters.

Because a body of existing studies examine the activity–cognition relationships, chapter 2 (Tomporowski) summarizes 17 existing reviews to identify and consolidate key findings and needed directions. The chapter also discusses methodological and design issues as well as theory development. Chapter 3 (Poon and Harrington) extends and integrates the theoretical positions posed in chapters 1 and 2. This chapter reviews similarities of research and postulated cognitive mechanisms in the aging-related and fitness-related literature.

The second part of this book, chapters 4 and 5, focuses on potential neurobiological and physiological mechanisms that intervene between exercise and cognition. Chapter 4 (Dustman and White) begins with a review of the impact of exercise on basic functional properties of the brain such as cerebral blood flow, neurotransmitter function, the oxidation of glucose, brain plasticity, and the interplay between the central nervous system and inhibition, which governs all behaviors. Chapter 5 (Holmes) focuses on the neurobiological systems' response to exercise. This chapter examines the brain's monoaminergic neurotransmitters—serotonin, norepinephrine, and dopamine system—because they are involved in the regulation of cognitive processes, mood states, and disorders. The chapter focuses on serotonergic projections of the raphe nuclei, the noradrenergic projections of the locus coeruleus, and the mesotelencephalic dopamine systems. It discusses the significance of recent research concerning the capacity for exercise to increase the synthesis of neurotrophic factors in the brain.

The third part of this book, chapters 6 through 11, provides advances in measurement designs and tools that could increase measurement sensitivity in exercise, fitness, and cognition research. Chapter 6 (Dishman) outlines available instruments that could measure physical activities in free-living and unsupervised settings. Chapter 7 (Cress) discusses models and instruments in assessing physical and functional performances in older adults. Chapter 8 (O'Connor) focuses on the indirect effects of exercise on cognition and highlights three hypotheses that exercise could affect secondary aging factors, which in turn facilitate cognition in old age. Chapters 9 and 10 focus on new physiological tools that could evaluate the direct facilitative effects of exercise on cognition. Chapter 9 (McCully & Bhambhani) examines tools in the assessment of brain blood flow, and chapter 10 (Miller) summarizes neuroimaging techniques that could be used to test neurobehavioral hypotheses of exercise and cognition. Finally, chapter 11 (Spirduso) summarizes and discusses the contents of this volume. It also introduces the contents of the second volume.

As noted earlier, volume I is not designed to be exhaustive. It is designed to introduce salient issues and reviews and to raise consciousness among researchers, students, policy makers, and the lay public of the importance of an active lifestyle on the mind as a person ages. This three-volume series can be used as an up-to-date research reference as well as a classroom textbook on exercise, cognition, and aging.

CHAPTER 1

National Blueprint: Increasing Physical Activity Among Adults 50 and Older: Implications for Future Physical Activity and Cognitive Functioning Research

Wojtek Chodzko-Zajko, PhD

In May 2001, a major national planning document was released in the United States in an attempt to develop a national strategy to increase physical activity among older individuals. The *National Blueprint: Increasing Physical Activity Among Adults Age 50 and Older* was developed with input from more than 60 individuals, representing 46 organizations with expertise in health, medicine, social and behavioral sciences, epidemiology, gerontology and geriatrics, clinical science, public policy, marketing, medical systems, community organization, and environmental issues (Armstrong, Sloan, Turner et al., 2001).

The *Blueprint* recognizes that a substantial body of scientific evidence indicates that regular physical activity can bring dramatic health benefits to people of all ages and abilities and that this benefit extends over the entire course of life. Increasingly, evidence indicates that physical activity offers one of the greatest opportunities to extend years of active independent life, reduce disability, and improve the quality of life for older persons.

However, despite a wealth of evidence about the benefits of physical activity for older persons, there has been little success in convincing older Americans to adopt physically active lifestyles. For example, in the United States, a recent report by the surgeon general estimated that between one-third and one-half of Americans over the age of 50 get no leisure-time physical activity at all (U.S. Surgeon General's Report, 1996). The numbers are even higher for older people in some groups, especially in older women where the percentage of sedentary individuals may be as high as 70 percent.

A major goal of the *Blueprint* was to identify the principal barriers to physical activity participation in older adults and to outline strategies for increasing physical activity levels throughout the population. The *Blueprint* identifies specific needs in the areas of research, home and community programs, workplace settings, medical systems, public policy and advocacy, and crosscutting issues. In this paper, Chodzko-Zajko, an author of the national planning document and chairman of the national coalition charged with advancing the *National Blueprint* agenda, summarizes some of the challenges identified in the *Blueprint* and considers the implications of the *Blueprint* for researchers working in the area of physical activity and cognitive functioning.

Benefits of Physical Activity for Older Adults

The *Blueprint* begins with a summary of the evidence supporting the health benefits of physical activity participation among seniors. Because physical activity has been defined in many different ways, the *Blueprint* adopts the World Health Organization's broad and inclusive definition of physical activity, which includes all movements in everyday life, including work, recreation, exercise, and sporting activities (World Health Organization, 1997).

The physiological benefits of participation in regular physical activity are now well established. Among the short-term benefits attributed to regular exercise are improved sleep (Brassington & Hicks, 1995), improved glucose regulation (Giacca et al., 1994), and increases in catecholamine activity (Richter & Sutton, 1994). Long-term adaptations to extended exercise participation include improved cardiovascular performance, increased muscular strength and endurance, enhanced flexibility and range of motion, decreased adiposity, and improved lipid status (Spirduso, 1995). Goldberg and Hagberg (1990) have suggested that the physiological responses of elderly adults to exercise training are similar to those experienced by younger individuals. The World Health Organization (WHO) (1997) has summarized the known physiological benefits of regular physical activity as follows:

Immediate Benefits

- Glucose levels: Physical activity helps regulate blood glucose levels.
- Catecholamine activity: Both adrenalin and noradrenalin levels are stimulated by physical activity.
- Improved sleep: Physical activity has been shown to enhance sleep quality and quantity in individuals of all ages.

Long-Term Effects

- Aerobic and cardiovascular endurance: Substantial improvements in almost all aspects of cardiovascular functioning have been observed following appropriate physical training.

- Resistive training and muscle strengthening: Individuals of all ages can benefit from muscle strengthening exercises. Resistance training can have a significant impact on the maintenance of independence in old age.
- Flexibility: Exercise that stimulates movement through a range of motion assists in the preservation and restoration of flexibility.
- Balance and coordination: Regular activity helps prevent or postpone the age-associated declines in balance and coordination that are a major risk factor for falls.
- Velocity of movement: Behavioral slowing is a characteristic of advancing age. Individuals who are regularly active can often postpone this age-related decline.

Physical activity can also have significant psychological consequences. There is now compelling evidence that regular exercise enhances psychological health and well-being. Among the short-term psychological benefits attributed to regular exercise are improved relaxation (Landers & Petruzzello, 1994), reduced stress and anxiety (Petruzzello et al., 1991), and improved mood state (Nieman et al., 1993). More long-term benefits include improved life satisfaction (Berger & Hecht, 1990), enhanced self-esteem and heightened self-efficacy (McAuley & Rudolph, 1995), and fewer mood state disturbances (O'Connor, Aenchbacher, & Dishman, 1993). In addition, there is a growing body of evidence to suggest that long-term participation in physical activity may affect a variety of cognitive processing functions. The WHO (1997) has recently summarized the known psychological benefits of regular physical activity as follows:

Immediate Benefits

- Relaxation: Appropriate physical activity enhances relaxation.
- Reduces stress and anxiety: There is evidence that regular physical activity can reduce stress and anxiety.
- Enhanced mood state: Numerous people report elevations in mood state following appropriate physical activity.
- General well-being: Improvements in almost all aspects of psychological functioning have been observed following periods of extended physical activity.

Long-Term Effects

- Improved mental health: Regular exercise can make an important contribution in the treatment of several mental illnesses, including depression and anxiety neuroses.
- Cognitive improvements: Regular physical activity may help postpone age-related declines in central nervous system processing speed and improve reaction time.

- Motor control and performance: Regular activity helps prevent or postpone the age-associated declines in both fine- and gross-motor performance.

- Skill acquisition: New skills can be learned and existing skills refined by all individuals regardless of age.

In addition to the noted physical and psychological benefits, physical activity participation also has a number of significant short- and long-term effects on a variety of sociocultural variables. For example, aging is associated with a need to adjust to changing roles and loss of roles. Because of factors such as death of friends and loved ones, retirement, financial hardship, ill health, and isolation, many older people are forced to relinquish systematically more and more of the roles that they consider to be a meaningful part of their identity (McPherson, 1990). Physical activity can be helpful in assisting older persons to adjust better to these role losses. Activity programs can provide seniors with the opportunity to widen their social networks, to stimulate new friendships, and to acquire positive new roles in their retirement (McPherson, 1990; 1994). The WHO (1997) summarizes the known sociocultural consequences of regular physical activity as follows:

Immediate Benefits

- Empowering older individuals: A large proportion of the older-adult population voluntarily adopts a sedentary lifestyle that eventually threatens to reduce independence and self-sufficiency. Participation in appropriate physical activity can empower older individuals and assist them in playing a more active role in society.

- Enhanced social and cultural integration: Physical activity programs, particularly when carried out in small groups and in social environments, enhance social and intercultural interactions for many older adults.

Long-Term Effects

- Enhanced integration: Regularly active individuals are less likely to withdraw from society and more likely to actively contribute to the social milieu.

- Formation of new friendships: Participation in physical activity, particularly in small groups and other social environments, stimulates new friendships and acquaintances.

- Widened social and cultural networks: Physical activity frequently provides individuals with an opportunity to widen available social networks.

- Role maintenance and acquisition of new roles: A physically active lifestyle helps foster the stimulating environments necessary for maintaining an active role in society as well as for acquiring positive new roles.
- Enhanced intergenerational activity: In many societies, physical activity is a shared activity that provides opportunities for intergenerational contact, thereby diminishing stereotypic perceptions about aging and the elderly.

Barriers to Physical Activity Among Older Adults

A major goal of the *Blueprint* was to identify some of the complex barriers that impede efforts to increase and maintain physical activity among older adults. The *Blueprint* recognizes that many factors impede physical activity among adults age 50 and older. The *Blueprint* identifies six categories of barriers that will need to be addressed in order to increase substantively physical activity levels throughout society. The barriers are as follows.

Research Barriers

There is a lack of guidance on what types and amounts of physical activity are needed for specific health outcomes. Few studies have examined strategies for achieving long-term increases in physical activity. Research findings are rarely translated into practical intervention strategies that can be widely incorporated into ongoing home and community settings.

Home and Community Barriers

Many neighborhoods and communities are poorly designed, unsafe, and engineered in a manner that discourages regular physical activity among older adults. Few models exist for an integrated community approach to enable physical activity. Community resources (senior centers, senior residences, community centers, neighborhoods and apartment units, schools, and places of worship) are often disconnected. Health organizations need to become more integrated with professionals in urban and community planning, transportation, recreation, and design in order to participate in developing strategies that will make communities more activity friendly. Also contributing to their lack of physical activity is the fact that many older adults do not know how to start a safe and proper home-based physical activity program. However, such knowledge may be needed because many older adults may be isolated and lack transportation to community facilities and programs for physical activity.

Workplace Barriers

Good economic models are needed that illustrate the cost effectiveness to employers of increasing physical activity among older adults. Employers may have concerns about liability (e.g., the liability implications if an employee gets hurt or becomes ill while participating in an on-site physical activity program or event). Little evidence exists about what programs are effective and what measurable outcomes are most persuasive to management (e.g., improved productivity, reduced health care costs, reduced absenteeism).

Medical Systems Barriers

Traditional medical education gives minimal attention to disease prevention. Training on physical activity is often a low priority. Health care professionals do not have adequate, tested, and appropriate age-specific patient education materials on physical activity for older patients. There is no effective, easy-to-use, evidence-based physical activity prescription protocol for health care professionals (similar to the "ask, advise, assess readiness to change, assist, and arrange follow-up" protocol used for tobacco cessation). Furthermore, medical professionals do not have information about making referrals to community resources; they often lack knowledge about quality programs, materials, and resources.

Public Policy Barriers

Public policy organizations that could support increased physical activity initiatives are fragmented into areas such as public health, transportation, housing, parks and recreation, senior citizens' issues, and health care reimbursement issues. No coalition or agency addresses these in a crosscutting manner. Not enough good economic models exist that illustrate the cost benefits of increasing physical activity among adults who are over the age of 50. Such models could be useful to policy makers in considering alternative investments in promoting physical activity among people 50 and older.

Marketing and Communications Barriers

Many of the messages and information about physical activity and exercise have been unclear, at times inconsistent, and confusing to older people as well as to the general population, health professionals, and policy makers. There is minimal marketing research to define the perceptions, beliefs, and concerns of people age 50 and older about physical activity and aging. Not enough effective messages to communicate information about physical activity have been developed and tested. These messages may need to take into account the continuum of health and functional status from healthy to frail adults.

Implications for Research
Into Physical Activity
and Cognitive Functioning

Before discussing the implications of the *National Blueprint* for research into physical activity and cognitive functioning, it is valuable to review the major research questions that have been identified and to summarize the status of research findings relative to each of these questions (Chodzko-Zajko & Moore, 1994).

There is a long tradition of research examining the impact of exercise and physical activity on the processing of information by the central nervous system. Because cognitive performance is known to decline significantly with advancing age, much of the literature on physical activity and cognition has focused on the study of these relationships in older individuals. Among the major cognitive processes that have been studied are memory, attention, perception, vigilance, problem solving, reaction time, movement time, digit symbol substitution. It is generally accepted that age-related changes in cognitive performance appear to be maximized for tasks that require rapid or attentionally demanding processing and are minimized for tasks that are more automatic or that can be performed at a self-paced rate (Chodzko-Zajko, 1991).

The literature on physical fitness, cognition, and aging has focused on three major questions:

1. Do highly fit older adults exhibit superior cognitive performance when compared with less fit individuals of the same chronological age?

2. Can relatively short-term increases in physical activity bring about meaningful cognitive changes in previously sedentary older adults?

3. By what mechanisms do physical activity and fitness influence cognitive performance in old age?

Unfortunately, little consensus has emerged within the physical activity and cognition literature with respect to either how to define physical activity and fitness or how best to measure them. Accordingly, it is often difficult to draw meaningful comparisons across studies when attempting to synthesize what is known about the physical activity–cognition relationship. Nonetheless, a number of general conclusions can be drawn.

Do highly fit older adults exhibit superior cognitive performance when compared with less fit individuals of the same chronological age?   With respect to the relationship between physical fitness and health and cognitive decline in old age, there is clear evidence that ill health and disease impair cognitive performance. For example, impaired cognitive processing has been shown to be associated with numerous disease states. Patients with Parkinson's disease perform less well than age-matched controls on complex reaction-time tasks, as do individuals who have clinical depression, schizophrenia, and manic-depressive psychosis. Similar relationships have also been observed in cardiovascular and circulatory pathology. These studies suggest that a variety of disease states may be associated with disruption in cognitive performance, and that these disruptions may be more pronounced in older-adult populations.

The data examining the relationship between good health and cognitive performance are less clear. Modest but reliable differences in processing speed have been observed between athletes and nonathletes as well as between highly fit and less fit subjects. The finding that physical fitness is associated with an enhancement in cognitive processing speed has been replicated many times. The association between physical fitness and cognitive performance appears to generalize to a variety of aerobic exercise activities, including racquetball, walking and jogging, swimming, and other activities. A number of factors appear to influence the magnitude of the relationship between physical fitness and cognitive performance. A general introduction of these factors and measures is described below. The impact of exercise and activities on these measures are reviewed in chapters 2 and 3.

Speed of Processing

Many reaction-time studies report significant differences between highly fit and less fit older adults with only a few exceptions. These findings suggest that when cognitive performance is evaluated by tasks in which processing speed is the principal dependent measure, the relation between physical fitness and cognitive performance is likely to be augmented (Chodzko-Zajko & Moore, 1994).

Task Complexity

Less is known about the relation between physical fitness and performance on more complex tasks in which qualitative rather than temporal aspects of cognition are evaluated (e.g. memory, problem solving, sustained attention, dual-task performance). A number of researchers have suggested that processing demand is an important factor in determining the magnitude of the relation between physical fitness and cognitive performance. When cognitive tasks are selected that require considerable processing demand, physical fitness effects are likely to be robust; whereas, fitness effects are likely to be smaller or nonexistent for less effortful cognitive tasks (Chodzko-Zajko & Moore, 1994).

Practice

Extended practice has the effect of reducing the magnitude of age effects in motor and cognitive performance research. The relationship between practice on a cognitive task and its sensitivity to physical fitness in unclear. Stones and Kozma (1989) found that fitness effects were greatest for novel, relatively unpracticed tasks and smaller for overlearned, highly practiced movements.

Level of Activity and Fitness

On first glance, one of the most obvious subject-related factors influencing the cross-sectional relationship between physical fitness and cognitive performance ought to be the magnitude of the fitness differences between highly fit and less fit groups. Unfortunately, there is little evidence against which to test such a "dose-dependent" relationship.

To summarize the cross-sectional data, there is now a growing body of evidence to suggest that physically active and fit older adults often process cognitive information more efficiently than less fit individuals of the same chronological age. It is clear that the relationship between physical fitness and cognition is highly task dependent. Physical fitness effects are most likely to be observed in tasks that require rapid or effortful cognitive processing and are less likely to occur in self-paced or automatic processing tasks. Because numerous tasks and subject-related factors can influence the relationship between fitness and cognition, extreme caution is warranted before making generalizations about the influence of physical fitness on cognitive performance.

Can relatively short-term increases in physical activity bring about meaningful improvements in cognitive performance in previously sedentary older adults? In the first study to examine the effect of exercise training on cognitive functioning, Dustman and colleagues (1984) randomly assigned sedentary adults to aerobic exercise strength and flexibility or nonexercise control groups and assessed the effect of four months of training on a battery of cognitive tests. Significant pre-to-post changes were observed in the aerobic exercise group for some cognitive tasks but not for others. Specifically, improvements were observed for critical flicker fusion, the digit symbol substitution scale of the Wechsler Adult Intelligence Scale, simple reaction time, and the Stroop task, whereas no changes were seen for choice reaction time, Culture-Fair IQ Test, or digit span.

However, several subsequent studies were unable to replicate these training effects. For example, Blumenthal and Madden (1988) subjected middle-aged and older adults to four to eight months of aerobic exercise, strength training, yoga, or sedentary living and examined pre-to-post changes in a variety of cognitive parameters. No evidence was found that aerobic exercise enhanced cognitive performance (Blumenthal & Madden, 1988). Similarly, Panton and colleagues (1990) randomly assigned 49 older adults (age 70-79) to aerobic exercise, strength training, and sedentary control groups and assessed changes in reaction time in response to the various treatments. Despite substantial improvements in aerobic capacity

(20 percent), no effects of aerobic exercise training on cognitive parameters were observed (Panton et al., 1990).

Hawkins, Kramer, and Capaldi (1992) assessed the effect of exercise training on cognitive performance using cognitive measures similar to those selected by Blumenthal and Madden (1988). Older adults were randomly assigned to 10 weeks of aerobic exercise or sedentary control regimens. Cognitive performance was assessed using both single- and dual-task procedures. Although neither group changed with respect to single-task performance, significant changes in dual-task performance were observed for the exercise but not the control group. Hawkins and colleagues noted that their dual-task paradigm was associated with significantly greater temporal demand. They suggested that this difference in time pressure caused their cognitive measures to be more attentionally demanding and thus more sensitive to the effects of exercise training.

In general, researchers have opted for training programs of four to eight months in duration, presumably because these are the minimum durations required to obtain reliable training effects on cardiovascular parameters. However, it is unclear why these durations should be considered sufficient for the manifestation of meaningful changes in cognitive behavior. No clear picture has emerged with respect to the effect of exercise on cognitive performance. Several well-controlled studies have successfully demonstrated improvement in cognitive performance following training, while others have not.

By what mechanism does physical fitness influence cognitive performance? Despite the wealth of studies that have examined the relation between physical fitness and cognitive performance, surprisingly little is known about the mechanisms by which exercise or physical activity might influence cognition. The following is a brief introduction of these hypotheses. Detailed examination of the aforementioned mechanisms is contained in chapter 4.

Cerebral Circulation Hypothesis

It has been proposed that chronic exercise maintains cerebrovascular integrity by enhancing oxygen transportation to the brain. McFarland (1963) demonstrated that cognitive declines observed in elderly subjects were similar to impairments seen in younger individuals under conditions of hypoxia. Subsequent studies were able to demonstrate small but significant improvements in cognitive performance following hyperbaric oxygen supplementation. Rogers, Meyer, and Mortel (1990) classified 90 elderly volunteers into three discrete activity groups: (1) currently working; (2) retired, high activity; and (3) retired, low activity. Cerebral blood flow was measured by the radioactive Xe inhalation method, and cognitive performance was assessed using a standardized cognitive screening examination. Individuals in the retired, low-activity group had lower cerebral blood flow, and these changes were associated with significant decrements in cognitive performance. Rogers and his colleagues (1990) concluded that individuals who retire and lead a sedentary lifestyle are at an increased risk of cerebrovascular disease with associated cognitive impairment. In summary, there is some circumstantial evidence to suggest that impaired cerebrovascular circulation is associated with accelerated cognitive decline. However, the effect of either physical fitness or short-term exercise training on this relationship has yet to be definitively established.

Neurotrophic Stimulation Hypothesis

It has long been suggested that prolonged activity may be associated with an amelioration of the severity of neural degeneration with advancing age. Prolonged physical activity is associated with increased brain weight in both primates and rats, and movement-enriched environments are associated with increased capillary growth as well as an increased number of dendritic connections. Research in humans has also shown that significant neural changes accompany advancing age. For the most part, the relationship between physical activity, aging, and central nervous system integrity has yet to be subjected to experimental test. In summary, evidence from animal models suggests that physical activity may be associated with a diminution of age-related degenerative changes in several neurological parameters. While there are theoretical reasons to believe that similar processes may be operating in humans, there is a shortage of empirical data in this area, and further research is needed before definitive conclusions can be drawn.

Neural Efficiency Hypothesis

It is now well established that advancing age is associated with predictable changes in both raw and computer-averaged electrophysiological responses. For example, older adults exhibit decreased electroencephalogram (EEG) alpha frequencies when compared with younger subjects. Similarly, auditory, visual, and somatosensory averaged evoked potentials (AEPs) also demonstrate reliable changes with advancing age. Dustman, Emmerson, Ruhling, and colleagues (1990) studied the electrophysiological responses of young (20-31 years) and older (50-62) adults who were divided into highly fit and less fit groups in accordance with their maximal oxygen consumption. Age and fitness effects were observed for a variety of EEG parameters including somatosensory evoked potentials, visual evoked potentials, and cortical coupling. Cognitive performance was better for young men than for older men and for highly fit than for less fit subjects. The authors concluded that physical fitness was associated with more efficient CNS processing. Thus, there is some evidence that high levels of fitness may be associated with a reduction in the magnitude of the age-related changes in electrophysiological parameters. Highly fit individuals appear to process information faster and more efficiently than less fit individuals of the same chronological age.

Research Implications of the *National Blueprint: Increasing Physical Activity Among Adults Age 50 and Older*

The *National Blueprint* was written for multiple audiences and addressed a wide variety of different aspects of the relationship between physical activity and quality of life in old age. Accordingly, not all of the barriers and strategies identified in the *Blueprint* directly affect research questions related to physical activity and cognitive functioning. However, a number of important issues are raised which are clearly relevant and should be considered by researchers working in this area. The final section of the paper considers some of the barriers and challenges identified in the *Blueprint* and reflects on their implications for cognition research.

• **Need for more translational research.** A key research barrier identified in the *Blueprint* is the observation that research findings are rarely translated into practical intervention strategies that can be widely incorporated into ongoing home and community settings. This is particularly true for research into the relationship between physical activity and cognitive functioning. To date, almost all research in this area has been restricted to highly controlled laboratory investigations. In these studies, physical activity has typically been restricted to rigidly controlled experimental protocols that are not always representative of the types of physical activity performed by older adults in the real world. Also, most studies have assessed cognitive performance on a battery of laboratory tasks, and little is known about whether improvements on these tasks will generalize to cognitive functioning in everyday life. If physical activity and cognitive functioning research is to continue to be a funding priority for federal agencies and private foundations, in addition to examining the underlying theoretical basis for the relationship, more attention will need to be paid to the practical implications of this work for the quality of life of individuals living in the real world.

• **Need for more specific information about the types and amounts of physical activity needed for specific cognitive outcomes.** Although a relationship between physical activity and cognitive functioning has been shown for several types of physical activity and many different aspects of cognitive processing, there has been almost no attempt to examine the dose-dependent nature of the relationship. No data exist with respect to how much physical activity is necessary for achieving a specific improvement on a specific cognitive task. Most studies have focused on the effect of cardiovascular exercise and a few others have examined the impact of resistance training, but almost no information is available about the specific mode, intensity, duration, and frequency of exercise necessary to result in clinically meaningful cognitive improvements.

• **Need for more studies examining the long-term impact of physical activity.** Cognitive decline with aging is a process that occurs over a number of decades, beginning in middle age and gradually accelerating thereafter. Most studies of physical activity and cognition have been restricted to interventions lasting four to eight months. While four to eight months may be an appropriate time scale for assessing physiological changes in response to exercise training, it is less clear that this is an appropriate time course for the assessment of the impact of activity on cognitive change in old age. More studies are needed that systematically examine the long-term impact of activity on cognitive integrity. Both longitudinal and epidemiological evidence is needed in order to examine these long-term effects.

• **Need for a more integrated approach to the study of active aging.** In recent years, a consensus has emerged among gerontologists that a key objective of intervention programs in older-adult populations is the preservation or restoration of acceptable quality of life (QOL). Although QOL is difficult to define precisely, most researchers agree that quality of life is dependent on a complex combination of factors, including physical health, psychological well-being, social satisfaction, and spiritual contentment. It is increasingly clear that physical activity alone is insufficient for the promotion of high QOL in old age. To age successfully, older persons will need to be not only physically active but also socially, intellectually, culturally, and (for many seniors) spiritually active.

There is an abundance of evidence that enriched intellectual and social environments have the potential to positively affect cognitive performance in old age. Numerous studies have examined the effect of cognitive training on cognitive processing in older adults. Somewhat surprisingly, to date, few studies have attempted to examine the combined effects of physical, intellectual, and social activity on cognitive performance. There is a clear need to develop research paradigms that can better integrate physical activity into the wider social, cultural, and economic context of active aging as a whole.

Conclusion

Within the area of research, it is clear that aging is a multifaceted process. In the future, research in this area is likely to become increasingly interdisciplinary and multidisciplinary in nature (Chodzko-Zajko, 2000).

Scientists from many different backgrounds and areas of specialization will need to join together to form collaborative research teams that can address the complex issues related to healthy and successful aging. In this paper, some of the challenges facing physical activity and cognitive-functioning researchers have been discussed. It seems clear that researchers working in this area will need to pay greater attention to the practical implications of their work for the quality of life of individuals living in the real world. They will need to provide more specific information about the types and amounts of physical activity necessary for achieving improvements on specific cognitive tasks. They will need to design and implement more studies that systematically examine the long-term impact of physical activity on cognitive integrity. Finally, they will need to adopt a more integrated approach to the study of active aging in which the combined effects of physical, intellectual, and social activity on cognitive performance are examined in order to better integrate physical activity research into the wider social, cultural, and economic context of active aging as a whole.

CHAPTER 2

Physical Activity, Cognition, and Aging: A Review of Reviews

Phillip D. Tomporowski, PhD

Questions concerning the relationship between physical activity and mental activity have been posed for centuries. Central to the philosophical framework of Western civilization is the dualistic view that human behavior can be explained in terms of processes of the body and processes of the mind. The specific relationship that exists between the body and mind has been a topic of debate, discussion, and writing for more than two centuries. The questions that have been formulated both by ancient thinkers and by modern scientists reflect the zeitgeist. The questions of contemporary researchers reflect particular epistemological frameworks. Researchers explore the relation between physical activity and cognition from different perspectives. Some researchers use frameworks that emphasize physiological processes, others focus on psychological processes, and others have interests in hormic and motivational processes. Scientists interpret data obtained from studies that examine the relation between physical activity and cognition, and their interpretations reflect these various frameworks or points of view.

This review has two goals. The first is to showcase the historical views of the last two decades of researchers who have examined studies and who have provided interpretations of those studies that assess the impact of physical activity training on mental processing and behavior. A literature search led to the identification of 17 review papers, which were separated into three groups. One group of reviews focuses on the relation between physical activity and mental health; another group focuses on exercise's effects on cognition; and the third group examines the interrelation among exercise, cognition, and aging factors.

The second goal of this review is to highlight two issues deemed critical to any systematic study of physical activity and its impact on aging. The first deals with methodological and research design issues, and the second addresses issues related to theory development. A number of specific research questions are posed and suggestions concerning future directions are then provided.

Critical Reviews

Historians provide numerous examples of the importance that has been placed on physical activity as a method to develop and maintain physical and mental health and mental ability. As early as the fourth century B.C., the Greek philosopher Xenophon promoted the importance of exercise as a means of staving off declines in mental prowess associated with growing older. Socrates and Plato also discussed the merits of vigorous physical activity as a way to maintain a clear mind. During the Renaissance, physical activity was prescribed to ameliorate the extravagant lifestyles of the wealthy. Likewise, Shadrach Ricketson, who is credited in 1806 with the first American text on preventive medicine, devoted an entire chapter to the importance of exercise for maintaining health and vigor throughout the life span. Interestingly, the value of exercise as a health-promoting vehicle had been voiced most vigorously during times when communities experienced wealth and stability and had available leisure time.

The wellness movement in the United States in the 1970s spawned a tremendous interest in physical activity as a method to promote physical and mental health. The merits of running and aerobic activity proselytized by Ken Cooper, Jim Fixx, and others led millions to begin exercise training with the conviction that physical activity is a curative with the potential to offset or postpone the aging-associated deterioration of the body and mind. Since that time, the putative benefits of exercise on mental processing and its ability to offset the impact of aging have been described in more than 1,000 magazine and health-promotion articles written for the general public.

The academic study of the effects of physical activity on mental processing can be traced back to research conducted more than a century ago. The majority of published studies, however, has been conducted over the past three decades, and several reviews of these studies have been conducted (see bibliography on pages 27 and 28). Three reviews stand apart from the others in the manner in which they organize and describe the studies reviewed, address core methodological issues, present theory-based explanations for empirical observations, and propose directions for research and theory development.

Folkins and Sime

Folkins and Sime's (1981) review was published at a time when the aerobic exercise and health movement was gaining momentum; the review was designed to address the impact of physical activity both on nonclinical and on clinical populations. The authors evaluated studies that assessed the effects of aerobic-type exercise on the cognition, perception, affect, behavior (work, sleep, social behavior), and personality of individuals without clinical syndromes. They also evaluated studies that employed physical fitness training as an intervention for such clinical conditions as depression, anxiety, alcoholism, and mental retardation.

Folkins and Sime concluded that methodological shortcomings and procedural artifacts of many of the studies evaluated made it difficult to make firm conclusions regarding a causal relationship between physical fitness training and cognition or mental health. Only about 15 percent of the studies reviewed met the criteria of a true experiment. Physical fitness training leads to improved mood, self-concept, and work behavior. The effects of exercise on cognition are not clear; however, there are data that suggest that cognitive performance is enhanced during and following physical activity. The Folkins and Sime (1981) review has served as the primary catalyst for much of the academic study of exercise and psychological process that has been conducted over the past two decades. The authors identify three theoretical approaches that researchers take to evaluate the relation between exercise and mental processes:

- A physiological viewpoint. This implies a direct physical causation for the psychological benefits of fitness training.

- A psychological viewpoint. Physical fitness improvements provide people with a sense of mastery and control over their behavior; these changes mediate enhanced cognitive functioning.

- A cognitively oriented viewpoint. Physical fitness training is a self-regulation process that enhances adaptive behaviors.

Plante and Rodin

This review was designed specifically as an update of Folkins and Sime's (1981) review. It focused primarily on studies that examined the effects of exercise among nonclinical populations. The researchers evaluated 38 studies that did not suffer from extensive methodological shortcomings. These studies were grouped into four areas: well-being and mood, personality and self-concept, physiological stress responsivity, and cognition.

Plante and Rodin (1990) concluded that exercise improves mood and psychological well-being (especially immediately following exercise), and it improves self-concept and self-esteem. Exercise appears to do little for personality functioning. There is little evidence that exercise alters stress responsivity or cognitive functioning.

The Plante and Rodin (1990) review stresses the need to evaluate separately the effects of acute bouts of exercise and the effects of chronic exercise interventions. The authors reiterate Folkins and Sime's (1981) views on the lack of methodological rigor that exists in many of the studies that have been conducted. However, there is a need to conduct research aimed at addressing the importance of engaging in exercise activity relative to factors that motivate someone to become an exerciser. It is difficult to determine if exercise improves psychological functioning, or if exercisers as a group tend to be more psychologically fit than nonexercisers. There is also a need to conduct follow-up evaluations to determine if psychological improvements attributed to exercise are maintained.

Morgan

A significant contribution to the study of the mental health benefits of physical activity was provided by William Morgan (1997) in the form of an edited, uniquely organized text. It provided a series of comprehensive reviews of empirical studies that assessed the effects of physical activity on such factors as depression (Martinsen & Morgan, 1997), anxiety (Raglin, 1997), self-esteem (Sonstroem, 1997), and overtraining (O'Connor, 1997). The text also included a series of reviews that addressed potential explanations for observed relations between physical activity and mental health. Exercise-produced changes in endorphin (Hoffmann, 1997), serotonin (Chaouloff et al., 1987), norepinephrine (Dishman, 1997), and thermogenic (Koltyn, 1997) levels on affect were evaluated. However, issues that relate specifically to the relation between physical activity and cognition were not addressed.

The contributions of Morgan's book, including the questions raised for future research, include a cogent overview of methodological issues that is particularly relevant to the assessment of physical activity and its effects on psychological variables, the evaluation of effects of exercise from the perspective of both basic and applied research. Attention is paid to the potential of exercise to produce both positive and negative outcomes. The book postulates that the consequences of exercise on mental health depend on the parameters of the training program.

The "dose-effect" relation between exercise and mental health is not known. It is unclear if there is a "threshold" effect; that is, does the dose-effect relation require a specific level of improvement to elicit a change in psychological functioning? Future research should address issues related to exercise mode, intensity, duration, preferred versus prescribed exercise, personalized prescription, and lifestyle versus traditional exercise prescription.

Physical Activity and Cognition

The hypothesis that aerobic exercise can serve as a vehicle to promote positive changes in affective states has received considerable empirical support. Indeed, Morgan (1997) suggests that "there is no further need for research or reviews dealing with the question of whether or not physical activity results in improved mood. There is compelling evidence supporting the efficacy of physical activity in the prevention and treatment of both physical and mental disorders" (p. 230). However, the evidence in favor of the effectiveness of exercise programs on changing cognitive functioning was less clear.

Two reviews, Gutin (1972) and McMorris and Graydon (2000), address directly the relation between exercise-induced arousal and cognitive performance. The notion that performance is associated with arousal level has long been a part of psychological research. The formulation of the Yerkes-Dodson law (1908), which hypothesizes an inverted U-shaped function between arousal and performance, figured prominently in early learning theory and has had an impact on modern theories of human performance.

Both of these reviews examined studies that were designed based on *a priori* predictions derived from theories that were grounded in the Yerkes-Dodson law. These studies are characterized by the repeated assessment of an individual's cognitive performance as his or her level of physical arousal increases as a direct function of exercise. Typically, exercise protocols include bouts of aerobic and anaerobic exercise that are relatively brief; most protocols last less than 20 minutes. Demonstration of an initial improvement in performance, followed by a decline in performance as arousal increases from a resting state, is taken as support for the Yerkes-Dodson law.

The authors concluded that the results of laboratory studies that attempt to link cognitive performance to specific levels of exercise-produced arousal are ambiguous. There are studies that provide clear evidence for an inverted U-shaped relation between arousal and cognitive performance, studies that provide only partial support for the relation, and still other studies that provide no support for the relation. Gutin (1972) concluded that the relation between exercise and performance may be negative, positive, or curvilinear, depending on the kind of task used. McMorris and Graydon (2000) concluded that exercise-induced arousal is limited to information-processing speed and has little influence on complex decision making.

Based on the review, Gutin proposed the implementation of research strategies that incorporate physiological, neuropsychological, and behavioral measures of exercise's effects on cognition. Also suggested were the utilization of the measures of participants' fitness status and the reevaluation of the concept of arousal and the incorporation of new theories of mental processing.

Three reviews focused on studies that examined the effects of acute bouts of exercise on cognitive performance. Acute exercise protocols result in the activation of the entire body and produce systemic changes in physiological functions such as cardiorespiration, endocrine function, and body temperature. In these studies, measures of cognitive performance are taken while an individual is in the process of exercising or shortly following the termination of exercise.

Weingarten

This review focused on studies that examined mental performance during and immediately following exercise. Weingarten (1973) concluded that physically fit individuals have a definite advantage over nonfit individuals when mental tasks are administered during or immediately after physiological stress. The advantage of physical fitness is not evidenced under normal conditions.

Tomporowski and Ellis

These authors classified 27 studies into three groups on the basis of the duration and intensity of the exercise protocol. Tomporowski and Ellis (1986) concluded that the data obtained from the studies reviewed failed to support the notion that exercise influences cognition.

Tomporowski

A review of 43 studies examined the effects of acute bouts of exercise on cognitive functioning. Studies were separated into one of three groups on the basis of the focus of the intensity and duration of the exercise protocols employed. One group focused on the construct of fatigue and studies that employed brief, maximal exercise protocols. A second group focused on the construct of arousal and studies that employed both maximal and submaximal exercise protocols of short duration. The third group focused on the effects of submaximal exercise protocols of relatively long duration.

Tomporowski (2003) concluded that moderate levels of aerobic, steady-state exercise facilitate specific stages of information processing. Exercise does not influence directly those operations involved in the initial stage of processing. Studies consistently fail to find systematic exercise effects on tasks that measure perceptual and sensory processing. However, exercise does influence the decision-making stage of information processing. Faster choice responses have been observed both on simple and complex tasks during and following exercise. In most cases, response speeds increase with no accompanying increase in error rates, suggesting that exercise is not simply altering participants' response criterion. Rather, exercise produces a condition during which individuals are able to perform both simple and complex tasks rapidly and efficiently.

Studies that employ tasks that measure response inhibition provide compelling evidence for exercise's influence on working memory. Acute bouts of exercise improve the ability to block irrelevant information and to select and respond to task-relevant information. Although exercise alters working-memory processes, it does not influence retrieval of information from long-term memory. Furthermore, exercise has clear effects on the response-preparation stage of information processing. The capacity to mobilize and to time movement patterns is enhanced during and following bouts of steady-state aerobic exercise. Intense anaerobic exercise does not impair cognitive function significantly; however, submaximal aerobic exercise that leads to dehydration does compromise both information processing and memory functions.

The author made three other conclusions regarding the effects of exercise on cognition. First, acute bouts of moderately intense exercise are hypothesized to function in a manner similar to that of psychostimulant drugs, which do not influence directly the computational processes that are involved in information processing. Rather, they produce changes in state processes that are responsible for the allocation of attentional resources. Second, the magnitude of acute exercise's effects on cognitive function is expected to interact with a variety of individual difference variables. Several of the studies reviewed reported that exercise's impact on performance depended on the participants' level of physical fitness or their level of experience. Finally, the conclusions drawn from empirical studies evaluated can be explained in the context of contemporary energetic models of cognition. These theories attempt to capture the relation among the components of the information-processing system, the allocation of energy that is involved in mental operations, and the guidance functions of executive processes.

Etnier, Salazar, Landers, Petruzzello, Han, and Nowell

This review examined the roles of both acute exercise interventions and chronic exercise interventions on cognitive functioning. Etnier and colleagues (1997) conducted a meta-analysis of 134 studies that evaluated the relation between exercise and cognitive function. They separately examined studies that examined exercise's acute effects and chronic effects on exercise. The results of the meta-analysis were used to test nine hypotheses generated from previous literature reviews.

The authors concluded that exercise has a small positive effect on cognition ($ES = 0.25$). However, the importance of this finding must be judged in light of subsequent analyses, which suggest that the impact of single bouts of aerobic exercise is limited only to improvements in participants' simple reaction time. The analysis identified a negative relation between acute exercise and participants' performance on tasks that measured either choice or discriminant reaction time.

Also, exercise appears to have a meaningful impact on cognition when it is administered as a chronic treatment to produce fitness gains. Further, the impact of exercise increases with training duration. However, the importance of this finding needs to be judged in light of numerous methodological flaws that exist in many studies. Furthermore, Etnier and colleagues (1997) determined that the age of the participants did not have a significant impact on the effect size generated by the meta-analysis.

In recent years, controversy has shifted from the question of whether there is a link between mind and body to the question of what the precise causal relationship is between the two components. Exercise's impact on cognition may be explained in terms of its impact on cerebral blood flow, modification of neurotransmitter systems, or structural changes in the brain.

Physical Activity, Cognition, and Aging

Throughout history, numerous methods have been proposed to stave off age-related declines in mental abilities. One method that has been consistently suggested to have ameliorative effects on mental processing is physical activity. In today's popular culture, involvement in physical activity is believed to offset declines in abilities associated with advancing age; articles in popular literature tout the beneficial effects of exercise. Some articles encourage older adults to participate in such physical activities as walking, swimming, and cycling. The commonsense belief that physical activity maintains one's general health has led to the development of various programs designed to improve abilities, prevent the onset of decline of abilities, and restore lost abilities.

Reviews of studies that examine the relation among exercise, cognition, and aging tend to fall on a continuum. At one end are reviews that address basic research questions, and at the other end are reviews that address applied research questions.

Spirduso

This classic review article focused on age-related changes in psychomotor speed and the impact that physical fitness has on psychomotor speed. The author evaluated a number of studies within several research domains considered to be relevant to understanding age-related changes in psychomotor speed. The areas reviewed included psychomotor performance of young and older adults who differed in level of physical fitness, the influence of physical fitness training on psychomotor speed, psychomotor speed with supplemental oxygenation, and psychomotor speed and cardiovascular disease.

The author concluded that many of the studies reviewed possessed methodological or design weakness. However, it appears that the psychomotor speed of fit young and older adults is faster than the speeds of their less fit age-mates, and that physical training programs result in the improvement of participants' response speeds. Furthermore, cardiovascular diseases compromise older adults' psychomotor speed, and supplemental oxygen can improve psychomotor functioning in some individuals.

Spirduso (1980) stated that the basis for fitness-related differences in psychomotor speed may be caused by such physiological mechanisms as cerebral blood flow, maintenance of the neural integrity of motor and somatosensory brain areas, and enhancement of brain neurotransmitter production. Furthermore, empirical evidence and theoretical supposition suggest that exercise modifies the brain structures that are involved in age-related slowing. Exercise may postpone psychomotor decline and have a significant impact on older adults' daily activities. Advances in the field will be spurred when greater attention is paid to physical and cognitive measurement.

Stones and Kozma

The main thrust of the review was to present various models that might explain the relation between physical activity and cognition. The authors contrasted the merits of three models. The health mediation model suggests that the prevention of ill health through exercise will help postpone disease states that have debilitating impacts on mental cognitive abilities. The moderator variable model suggests that lifelong exercising postpones or arrests age changes by maintaining processes that underlie performance ability (e.g., brain systems). The functional age model suggests that chronic exercise has generalized benefits for the organism, but it does not assume that the aging process itself is affected by exercise. The effects of chronic exercise can be described as tonic, meaning that vigor and vitality are restored to the performance of a range of functions. Health activities, such as exercise, contribute independently to overall capability to function.

The authors assess the empirical support for each of these models by drawing on published research and an extensive evaluation of two of their own studies designed to test the validity of the functional age model. They concluded that there was minimal support for either the mediation model or the moderator model. Furthermore, the studies reviewed provide support for the functional age model and the hypothesis that chronic exercise has a generalized effect across both physical and psychological domains. Exercise helps compensate for age deterioration by bolstering functional capability (e.g., vigor and vitality). Also, the improvement in cognitive performance is probably due to changes in brain oxygen transport capabilities brought about by exercise.

Stones and Kozma (1988) also asserted that physical activity can influence cognitive performance in two ways. Chronic exercise produces a generalized, or tonic, effect on functional capability that can be engendered at any point throughout the life span. Second, the repetitive nature of exercise leads to overpractice of specific motor movement patterns that are resistant to aging effects. The tonic and overpractice effects (TOPE) model provides a framework for assessing the dual nature of chronic exercise training.

Emery, Burker, and Blumenthal

This review reports the results of studies selected from a number of research domains. Emery, Burker, and Blumenthal (1991) assessed the impact of acute bouts of aerobic exercise on mood and cognitive functioning and the impact of chronic exercise on older adults' personality, mood, and cognitive functioning. The authors concluded that data from studies that examined the acute effect of exercise are scarce, and those that are available are difficult to interpret because of methodological problems. Also, the few studies that are available suggested that chronic exercise influences personality functioning.

The results of several studies conducted to evaluate the impact of chronic exercise on older adults' mood states are inconsistent. A number of studies were conducted during the 1980s and early 1990s that examined the effects of chronic exercise programs on older adults' cognitive performance (Blumenthal & Madden, 1988; Blumenthal et al., 1989; Blumenthal et al., 1991; Dustman et al. 1984; Dustman, Emmerson, Ruhling, et al. 1990; Madden, Blumenthal, Allen, & Emery, 1989; Panton et al. 1990). The results of these studies are mixed. Comparisons among these studies are made difficult by the differences that exist in research methodology, statistical analyses, and outcome measures. No intervention studies have been conducted that assess the impact of physical fitness training on neuropsychological performance of older adults following an acute bout of exercise. Furthermore, there have been no studies conducted of cardiovascular reactivity among older adults, which is a promising area for research in aging.

Therefore, more systematic studies need to be conducted; however, the boundaries of these studies should be expanded. Researchers should incorporate measures of self-perceptions of both emotional and physical status, indices of psychosocial functioning, self-esteem, and personal efficacy. Researchers will also need to address the issue of noncompliance or participant dropout.

Dustman, Emmerson, and Shearer

The authors examined studies investigating animal research that involved physical activity training of rodents and dogs, cross-sectional research that compared measures of the cognitive and neuropsychological processes of individuals who exercise with those of sedentary individuals, and intervention research that assessed the effects of aerobic exercise training on older adults' cognitive and neuropsychological processes.

Dustman, Emmerson, and Shearer (1994) concluded that research conducted with animals provided compelling evidence that improvements in aerobic fitness are linked to enhanced behavioral and neurobiological functioning. Aerobically fit animals differ from less fit animals on measures of acetylcholine, dopamine, norepinephrine, serotonin, and gamma-aminobutyric acid (GABA). Exercise participation beginning in middle age and continuing into old age can offset declines in neural integrity that typically occur during aging, both in animals and in humans.

Cross-sectional research indicated a strong positive association between physical activity level and cognitive performance. Physically active individuals consistently perform better on tests that demand speeded performance than those who are sedentary. The benefits of physical fitness are seen most clearly on cognitive tasks that provide measures of mental flexibility. However, intervention studies have not consistently demonstrated cognitive–neuropsychological improvements following exercise training.

The authors further concluded that converging evidence taken from three areas of research suggested that physical activity is associated with fundamental changes in the brain function, and that these improvements have an impact on age-related changes in mental processing. The results obtained from studies involving animal research, although compelling, must be evaluated with caution. It is not known if the exercise-based neuroanatomical changes found in animals generalize to the functioning of older adults. Research in the field will benefit from taking a life span approach.

The role of response inhibition across the life span may provide a way to assess physical fitness effects on adaptive behavior. Response inhibition involves the control of thought and action. It is known that inhibitory efficiency decreases with aging. The brain's capacity to benefit from physical activity is reduced with aging. Thus, the sooner exercise interventions are made a part of one's lifestyle, the greater the impact they will have on forestalling age-related changes in cognition.

Chodzko-Zajko and Moore

Chodzko-Zajko and Moore (1994) reviewed cross-sectional studies that examined the differences between highly fit and less fit older adults' cognitive performance and reviewed intervention studies that examined the effect of physical fitness training on older adults' cognitive functioning. These studies were evaluated in terms of a resource theory of attention that hypothesizes that cognitive processes can be distributed along an automatic-to-effortful continuum. Tasks that require the allocation of attentional resources are viewed as effortful, while tasks that are only minimally dependent on attentional resources are viewed as automatic. Theorists who employ resource models of cognition suggest that aging is associated with a reduction of attentional reserve.

The authors concluded that data obtained in cross-sectional research suggested that the cognitive functions of physically fit older adults are more efficient than those of their less fit peers. The relation between fitness and cognitive performance appears to be task dependent. Data obtained from intervention studies failed to support the view that physical activity training results in clinically significant improvements in cognition. Physical fitness effects are most likely to be observed in tasks that require rapid or effortful cognitive processing and are less likely to occur in self-paced tasks. There are several potential mechanisms by which physical activity may directly or indirectly influence older adults' cognitive processes. These include improvements in cerebral oxygenation, neurotrophic stimulation, and neural efficiency.

Kramer and Colleagues

Presented as a chapter in an edited text, and while not developed as a review of the literature, this work provided a significant contribution to the literature. Kramer, Hahn, and colleagues (2002) described a major research study that involved the assessment of the effects of a six-month physical fitness training program on 124 sedentary but healthy older adults. A cognitive test battery was constituted on the basis of the hypothesis that improvements in aerobic fitness would be associated with selective improvements in cognitive functions that involve executive control processes such as coordination, inhibition, schedule planning, and working memory. The exercise program resulted in improvements on the majority of cognitive tasks predicted to reflect executive control processes.

The authors concluded that the data obtained do not support the resource allocation hypothesis. Physical activity produces its beneficial effects on cognition through its impact on executive control processes. It was observed that the performance of subjects who exercised improved on tasks that require the capacity to retain and manipulate information in working memory, to perform two or more tasks concurrently, to switch rapidly between two tasks, and to inhibit prepotent responses. No attempts have been made to examine the relation among aerobic fitness, cognition, and brain function and structure. There is strong support from data obtained from neuroimaging studies that implicate the role of frontal-lobe processes and executive control. The development of nonintrusive neuroimaging techniques, such as functional magnetic resonance imaging (fMRI), provides a unique opportunity to examine fitness effects on both the brain and mind.

Two reviews, Shephard and Leith (1990) and Boutcher (2000), have examined the exercise literature with a view toward its application to health programs that are designed for older adults. Shephard and Leith (1990) provided a description of age-related changes in physiological, psychological, and emotional systems. They then addressed the impact that physical activity training has on each of these systems. The effects of habitual exercise's impact on normal and pathological aging processes were also assessed.

The authors concluded that physical activity training modifies anxiety and depression states. Habitual exercise may result in physiological and psychological hardiness. The effects of physical training programs on individuals with pathology are unclear. There is increasing evidence that habitual physical activity can improve cognitive function in older adults.

Exercise training programs must be designed to meet the needs of the individual. This is particularly true given possible interactions between medication and exercise. Particular efforts must be made to better understand compliance and adherence issues. This is especially true of individuals with pathological disorders.

Boutcher (2000) placed the major emphasis of his review on the effect that aerobic fitness has on the cognitive performance of older adults from nonclinical populations. The organization, presentation, conclusions, and discussion of the studies reviewed were similar to those presented by Chodzko-Zajko and Moore (1994). Boutcher concluded that the beneficial effects of habitual physical activity can be linked to changes in cerebral circulation, neurotrophic stimulation, and neural efficiency. Psychosocial processes linked to performance in exercise programs may facilitate older adults' level of motivation and contribute to cognitive-task improvement. There is a need for exercise scientists to collaborate with gerontological researchers. Randomized controlled trials must ensure that exercise training is sufficient to produce measurable improvements in physiological function.

ADDITIONAL REVIEWS

The following is a bibliography of reviews on exercise, activities, cognition, and aging not covered in this chapter. The reviews are clustered as published up to 1981, in the 1980s, and in the 1990s.

Reviews up to 1981

- Browman, C.P. (1981). Physical activity as a therapy for psychopathology: A reappraisal. *Journal of Sports Medicine, 21,* 192-197.
- Clarke, H.H. (1958). Physical fitness benefits: A summary of research. *Education, 78,* 460-466.
- Ismail, A.H. (1972). Integrated development. In J.E. Kane (Ed.), *Psychological aspects of physical education and sport.* London: Routledge.
- Layman, E.M. (1972). The contribution of play and sports to emotional health. In J.E. Kane (Ed.), *Psychological aspects of physical education and sport.* London: Routledge.
- Morgan, W.P. (1974). Exercise and mental disorders. In A. Ryan & F. L. Allman, Jr. (Eds.), *Sports medicine.* New York: Academic Press.
- Powell, R.R. (1975). Effects of exercise on mental functioning. *Journal of Sports Medicine & Physical Fitness, 15,* 125-131.

(continued)

(continued)

Reviews of the 1980s

- Doan, R.E., & Scherman, A. (1987). The therapeutic effect of physical fitness on measures of personality: A literature review. *Journal of Counseling & Development, 66,* 28-36.

- Hale, R.E., & Travis, T.W. (1987). Exercise as a treatment option for anxiety and depressive disorders. *Military Medicine, 152,* 299-302.

- Martinsen, E.W. (1989). The role of aerobic exercise in the treatment of depression. *Stress Medicine, 3,* 93-100.

- Oberman, A. (1984). Healthy exercise. *Western Journal of Medicine, 141,* 884-871.

- Phelps, J.R. (1987). Physical activity and health maintenance: Exactly what is known? *Western Journal of Medicine, 146,* 200-206.

- Ransford, C.P. (1982). A role for amines in the antidepressant effect of exercise: A review. *Medicine & Science in Sports & Exercise, 14,* 1-10.

- Rippe, J.M., Ward, A., Porcari, J.P., & Freedson, P.S. (1988). Walking for health and fitness. *Journal of the American Medical Association, 259,* 2720-2724.

- Sachs, M.L. (1982). Exercise and running: Effects on anxiety, depression, and psychology. *Humanistic Education & Development, 21,* 51-57.

- Simons, A.D., McGowan, C.R., Epstein, L.H., Kupfer, D.J., & Robertson, R.J. (1985). Exercise as a treatment for depression: An update. *Clinical Psychology Review, 5,* 553-568.

- Sonstroem, R.J. (1984). Exercise and self-esteem. *Exercise & Sports Science Review, 12,* 123-155.

- Taylor, C.B., Sallis, J.F., Needle, R. (1985). The relation of physical activity and exercise to mental health. *Public Health Reports, 100,* 195-202.

Reviews of the 1990s

- Arent, S.M., Landers, D.M., & Etnier, J.L. (2000). Effects of exercise on mood in older adults: A meta-analytic review. *Journal of Aging & Physical Activity, 8,* 407-430.

- Kramer, A.F., Hahn, S., & McAuley, E. (2000). Influence of aerobic fitness on the neurocognitive function of older adults. *Journal of Aging & Physical Activity, 8,* 379-385.

- Thomas, J.R., Landers, D.M., Salazar, W., & Etnier, J. (1994). Exercise and cognitive function. In C. Bouchard, R.J. Shephard, & T. Stephens (Eds.), *Physical activity, fitness, and health: Consensus statement* (pp. 521-529). Champaign, IL: Human Kinetics.

Inplications for Aging Research

Advances in understanding the effect that exercise training has on older adults' cognitive function will be realized when investigators employ research designs that avoid the methodological and procedural shortcomings that plague prior studies.

Methodological Issues

Virtually every review evaluated made a plea for more studies with adequate research design. Folkins and Sime (1981) reported that only about 15 percent of the studies they reviewed met the standards of a true experiment. Similar percentages are reported in other reviews. More recently, Etnier and colleagues (1997) identified 200 studies that examined exercise's effects on cognitive function, and they also addressed the serious design flaws present in many studies. They pointed out that support for the view that exercise benefits cognitive function comes primarily from cross-sectional and correlational studies, which do not provide a basis for establishing a causal relationship between exercise and cognition. The results obtained in these studies may be due to a wide variety of factors other than exercise, such as lifestyle choice, level of education, and socioeconomic status. Further, intervention studies are not immune to methodological problems. Their meta-analysis revealed that the effect sizes for chronic exercise studies were greater when participants were allowed to self-select a treatment condition than when participants were randomly assigned to a treatment.

Morgan (1997) provided an excellent review of issues that are central to physical activity research. He described how research outcomes can be influenced by such variables as participant and experimenter expectancies, demand characteristics, and the Hawthorne effect. Addressed also are several design issues that can make difficult the interpretation of research outcomes, such as sample size, statistical analysis approaches, and test selection. Test selection was identified by many reviewers as a particularly vexing problem. For example, Etnier and colleagues (1997) reported that 106 different cognitive tests were used in the studies they evaluated.

Procedural Issues

A number of factors either mediate or moderate the effect of exercise on older adults' cognitive function. It will important for researchers to isolate and evaluate the interactive effects of these variables.

Chronic Versus Acute Exercise Interventions

Reviewers tend to categorize exercise interventions into two types: acute and chronic. There are reviews that examine only acute effects or only chronic effects of exercise on mental processing. The separation of these two research approaches may make sense when conducting a review of the exercise literature. At some point, however, it will be essential to evaluate the impact of acute bouts of exercise within the context of chronic exercise interventions. Researchers who examine exercise's acute effects on cognition tend to recruit participants, conduct a few sessions during which the level of exercise intensity and duration is manipulated, then release the participant to the wild, never to be seen again. Researchers who examine exercise's chronic effects tend to recruit a sample of participants, obtain preexercise measures of psychological and physiological function, turn the participants over to exercise leaders for a prescribed duration, then obtain postexercise measures of physical and mental function. Presently, there are no studies that examine the impact of individual exercise bouts that take place in the context of long-term training.

There is compelling evidence that brief bouts of exercise enhance affect and cognitive function. Little is known, however, about how repeated bouts of exercise affect these variables. Researchers who track the impact of individual exercise sessions within long-term exercise programs may provide data that are critical to understanding the relation not only between exercise and cognition but also between exercise and participant compliance and attrition.

Follow-Up Evaluations

The study reported by Kramer, Hahn, and colleagues (2002) provided clear evidence for the positive effect of aerobic exercise training on the specific cognitive functions of older adults. It is hoped that studies designed to replicate the findings of this study will include follow-up evaluations to assess the long-term benefits of aerobic exercise training.

Issues of Individual Differences

Once over the hurdle of establishing that chronic physical activity has a salutary effect on cognition, we can begin to examine individual differences and the effects of exercise on cognition. These individual difference factors include: initial level of physical fitness, history of exercise training, history of skill development and expertise, personality, and presence of disease states (e.g., Alzheimer's disease and Parkinson's disease).

Theoretical Issues

The observations made by Folkins and Sime (1981) continue to hold true. The explanations provided by researchers for exercise's effects tend to be of three types: physiological, psychological, and cognitive. The review of reviews conducted here suggests that considerable progress has been made in each of these areas over the past two decades.

Physiological Approach

It is clearly the case that the zeitgeist has shifted toward physiological explanations for exercise's effects on human behavior. The roles of brain structures and functions have been discussed in relation to mental health, affect, and cognition. Many reviewers look forward to the application of technological advances to elucidate the mechanisms that account for cognitive and behavioral changes that accompany improvements in fitness and health.

Psychological Approach

Several researchers suggest that we not lose sight of the fact that exercise's impact on mental health and cognition will ultimately depend on an interaction between the individual and his or her environment. Progress in the field will be made through multidisciplinary research studies that evaluate the impact of lifestyle changes in health-promoting behaviors, only one of which is physical activity.

Cognitive Approach

Several theory–based reviews of studies have been published recently. These theories include attentional resource theory (Chodzko-Zajko & Moore, 1994), executive control theory (Kramer, Hahn, et al., 2002) and cognitive-energetics theory (Tomporowski, 2002). Several reviewers note that theory-driven research will lead to a better understanding of body–mind connections than the atheoretical approach that typifies much of the research in the field. However, some have expressed words of caution. It will be important for theories of cognition to fit into more general theories of human behavior that address life span issues.

Spirduso provides a framework for evaluating the complex relations that exist among health, fitness, and cognitive function. As noted in chapter 11 of *Physical Dimensions of Aging* (Spiriduso, 1995), cognitive function is the result of both primary aging factors and secondary aging factors. Primary aging factors that affect cognition include cerebrovascular change, neurotransmitter depletion or malfunction, brain morphological changes, and neuroendocrine function deterioration. Secondary aging factors include disease, accident, and environmental hazards. Health behaviors that can modify both primary and secondary aging factors include diet, absence of drug abuse, controlled stress, sleep, and exercise.

Future Directions

If the question, "Does physical activity influence cognitive function?" were posed to researchers only a few years ago, the answer would have been a weak "maybe." If the question were "Does physical activity influence older adults' cognitive function?" the answer would have been an even weaker "maybe" (Thomas, Landers, Salazar, & Etnier, 1994). Indeed, a meta-analysis conducted by Etnier and her associates, published as recently as 1997, suggests that acute bouts of exercise may impede cognitive performance, and the impact of chronic exercise training is modest.

Recent research and evaluation of the exercise literature lead to a different interpretation of the relation between exercise and cognitive function. Today it can be stated firmly that yes, indeed, exercise, both acute and chronic, facilitates specific aspects of cognitive functioning, and exercise interventions do facilitate specific aspects of older adults' cognitive functioning. Further, the specific cognitive processes that are enhanced by exercise play important roles in one's daily life and are critical to adaptive functioning.

Supporting the basic assumption that physical activity influences cognitive function leads to a number of important questions (Bouchard, Shephard, & Stephens, 1994; Boutcher, 2000). Some of these questions are:

- What is the dose-response relationship between exercise and cognition? Is there a threshold of physical fitness change that is required to promote improvements in cognitive function?
- Are there specific types of cognitive processes that are more sensitive than others to exercise's effects?
- Are the benefits engendered by exercise similar across the life span?
- What happens to the cognitive performance of those individuals who stop exercising?
- What are the mechanisms by which exercise influences cognitive functions?
- What types of exercises are most effective in promoting improvements in cognitive function?

CHAPTER 3

Commonalities in Aging- and Fitness-Related Impact on Cognition

Leonard W. Poon, PhD, and Carol Ann Harrington, MS

Chodzko-Zajko (chapter 1) and Tomporowski (chapter 2) reviewed empirical, methodological, and theoretical issues that pertained to this question: Do highly fit older adults exhibit superior cognitive performance when compared with less fit individuals of the same age? Both authors agreed that empirical data provided a positive *yes* to the question. Tomporowski outlined a number of competing theoretical positions relating to the loci of impact of exercise, activities, or fitness on cognition. The goal of this chapter is to integrate and summarize theoretical positions posed in chapters 1 and 2 and examine commonalities in the impact of aging- and fitness-related differences on cognitive functioning. The primary question posed in this chapter is whether the lack of fitness in old age is a risk factor for lower cognitive health; the reverse side of the question is whether maintenance of fitness is a protective factor.

Studies of fitness, cognition, and aging have theoretical, clinical, and ecological validity. Changes and differences in cognitive aging have long been a focus of research in the experimental psychology of aging (Poon, 1980, 1985; Salthouse, 1992, 1999). From an ecological perspective, the fear of losing one's memory is one of two major concerns of those who are growing old (Lowenthal & Berkman, 1967); the other concern is the loss of energy. Health care workers are quick to report that their older adults frequently worry that benign incidences of forgetfulness portend signs of Alzheimer's disease (Bowles, Obler, & Poon, 1989). The demonstration of noninvasive techniques that could provide a protective measure toward cognitive maintenance in aging would be a significant contribution to public health, especially if these interventions were effective over time. Unfortunately, research to date on exercise intervention has not been promising (see reviews in chapters 1 and 2).

Successful intervention would depend on identifying the underlying causes of cognitive decline. As reviewed in chapter 2, postulations are plentiful on the loci of impact of exercise on cognition; however, consensus has been elusive. To fulfill the vision of recommending fitness and exercise as a protective factor for cognitive decline, it is imperative to identify the underlying causes as to why and how highly fit older adults tend to perform at a higher level cognitively compared to less fit adults of the same age.

The Search for Underlying Mechanisms

Inspection of the literature seems to indicate that parallel approaches are employed to examine underlying mechanisms of cognitive differences between younger and older adults and highly fit and less fit adults. Three major lines of research and hypothesized theories in aging and fitness are reviewed in this chapter. They are attentional resource reduction theories, frontal system deficit theories, and generalized decrement theories.

Attentional Resource Reduction Theories

Attention is defined as the capacity or energy to support cognitive processing (Plude & Hoyer, 1985). Attention is viewed as being limited in resource or capacity. It is a necessary precursor to support and direct information processing that underlies perception, memory, decision making, and other cognitive processes. Four common types of attention processes are divided, switching, sustained, and selective. This perspective suggests that attentional resources are reduced in old age, which in turn reduces the efficiency in which cognitive processes are executed (Craik & Byrd, 1982; Hasher & Zacks, 1979; Wright, 1981).

In a review of memory and aging, Craik noted the following: "One of the clearest results in the experimental psychology of aging is the finding that older subjects are more penalized when they must divide their attention, either between two sources, input and holding or holding and responding" (1977, p. 391). Within this view of cognitive aging, Craik and Lockhart (1972) postulated that older adults' cognitive performances are negatively related to levels or effort of processing. Older adults are restricted in cognitive resources to process more effortful task demands.

Along a similar line of reasoning, Hasher and Zacks (1988) offer an alternative view: Age-related decrements in the inhibitory control mechanisms of cognition allow irrelevant information to enter working and secondary memory, thus compromising retrieval. McDowd and Craik (1988) and Salthouse, Rogan, and Prill (1984) concluded that disproportional deficits in the cognitive performance of older adults (a task complexity phenomenon) exist in divided attention in all but the simplest tasks (Somberg & Salthouse, 1982). Similar findings were reported in attention switching, selective attention, and sustained attention and aging (McDowd & Birren, 1990).

Concurring with the findings of these aging studies, the task complexity phenomenon was confirmed by Chodzko-Zajko and Moore (1994) in a review of studies with highly fit and less fit older adults (see chapters 1 and 2). Although highly fit and less fit older adults do not differ in their ability to perform automatic tasks, the difference is profound in effortful tasks. Lower cognitive performances of less fit adults could be explained by the resource theory of attention along the automatic-to-effortful continuum. The results suggested that the lower levels of attentional resources of the less fit adults were more apparent in tasks requiring higher cognitive performances.

Two studies illustrate this complexity effect. One of the first studies that elucidated cognitive differences between active lifelong and novice young and older racquetball players was performed by Spirduso (1975). She examined simple and discrimination reaction times of young (20-30 yrs) and older players (50-70 yrs). One group of each age had played racquetball at least three times a week for three years, and one group of each age was sedentary. She found that although there was no difference between simple and discrimination reaction times among young racquetball players, the older racquetball players far surpassed their sedentary counterparts on both simple- and discriminating-movement reaction times. The significant reaction time differences ranged from 23 to 68 percent between the fit and sedentary individuals. This study was replicated by Spirduso and Clifford (1978) to show the differential effects of age and activities (or level of expertise) on reaction times varying in cognitive loads and task demands.

Another example of manipulating the effects of task demands on cognition among active and inactive older adults was conducted by Abourezk (1989). The study used a more complicated dichotic listening task to ascertain the impact of exercise on cognition on 10 active and 10 inactive males from 50 to 70 years of age. The groups did not differ in digit comprehension when digits were presented monoaurally. They also did not differ when the digits were presented dichotically but the subjects were instructed to attend to only one ear. However, the active group was twice as efficient compared to the inactive group when digits were presented dichotically, although subjects were instructed to report digits presented to either ear. Thus, both groups were equally adept at hearing and understanding the digits in both ears and could selectively attend to one ear. However, the active group was twice as successful when the cognitive task was made more difficult by not specifying to which ear the digits would be presented.

Frontal System Deficit Theories

This class of theories focuses on the neuropsychological functioning of the frontal system in aging. A significant amount of research has been devoted to isolating biological correlates of cognitive aging (Ingram, 1988; Albert & Kaplan, 1980). It is known that age-related changes occur in the central nervous system. For instance, senile plaques and neurofibrillary tangles are found in greater concentrations in older compared to younger adults. Alterations in neuronal metabolism, such as changes in concentration of transmitter substances, have been widely reported for years. An important research question was whether these biological changes were related to generalized or specific changes in cognition among older adults.

Much of the extant knowledge about brain–behavior relationships has been derived from a comparison of brain-damaged patients to age-matched controls. Patterns of neuropsychological tests have shown that cognitive performances of normal elders are different from patients with diffuse brain damage. For example, Overall and Gorham (1972) administered the Wechsler Adult Intelligence Scale (WAIS) to men between the ages of 45 and 84, some of whom were healthy and some of whom were diagnosed with chronic brain disease. A multiple discriminant analysis on subtest scores revealed that the performances of normal controls did not resemble the performances of those with brain damage.

Similarly, Goldstein and Shelly (1975) administered the Halstead-Reitan Neuropsychological Test Battery to a group with diffuse brain damage and to healthy controls and found similar results. These well-cited studies have shown that aging is not equated with brain damage. However, specific neurological loci, such as the one that is found in the frontal area, are found to be associated with cognitive aging (Albert & Kaplan, 1980).

Studies in the last four decades were conducted to isolate unique neuropsychological correlates of cognitive aging (see reviews by Albert & Kaplan, 1980; Royall, Palmer, Chiodo, & Polk, 2004; and Royall et al. in volume II of this series). The majority of these frequently cited investigations focused on age-related differences in arousal and attention as well as visuospatial performances. For example, with aging, lower responses were found in the autonomic nervous system (e.g., reduced galvanic skin response in a vigilance task [Surwillo, 1966]) and central nervous system (e.g., small, late P300 components of average evoked electromyographical potential to cognitive processing, [Schenkenberg, 1970]).

In a classic study, Tecce (1978), using an average evoked potential distraction paradigm, found that older adults compared to younger controls were not able to shift attentional set, and this performance difference was evident in evoked potential in the frontal but not parietal area. Many of the findings supporting the attention deficit theories described earlier in this chapter also support the notion that an intact frontal system is needed in order to adequately perform attention-related tasks.

Further research reveals that an intact frontal system is needed in order to perform executive control, attention switching, and attention-sharing tasks such as planning, scheduling, task coordination, inhibition, and working memory associated with everyday life (Royall et al., 2004). Executive control was found to be lower in early childhood and older adulthood

(Cepeda, Kramer, & Gonzalez de Sather, 2001) and could be improved with practice (Mayr, Spieler, & Kliegl, 2001). Evidence from neuropsychological and neurobiological studies, along with data comparing aging and brain pathologies, supports the hypothesis that the frontal system makes an important contribution to age-related differences in cognitive processes.

Kramer and his colleagues (Cepeda, Kramer, & Gonzalez de Sather, 2001; Kramer, Hahn, & Gopher, 1999) have done extensive work on executive control functions and aging. Kramer's laboratory was also one of the first to hypothesize that executive control functions gain the largest fitness-induced benefits for older adults (Colcombe & Kramer, 2003; Kramer & Willis, 2002; Kramer, Hahn, & McAuley, 2000; also see chapter 2). This pioneering work has provided persuasive support for the frontal system deficit theories in pointing to this system as the primary locus in which aging-related cognitive deficits are found and also the locus in which fitness appears to exert its greatest influence.

Generalized Decrement Theories

An "intellectual tension" exists among cognitive-aging psychologists who postulate that cognitive aging is pervasive throughout the information processing system and those who suggest that the locus is specific to a process (such as the executive control functions). Earlier work has reported stage-specific decrements in that primary and tertiary memory suffer relatively small aging decrements, while secondary and working memory suffer profound deficits (Craik, 1977; Poon, 1985).

Similarly, stage-specific proponents suggest that automatic tasks are subject to minimal aging effects, while effortful tasks experience greater losses (Craik & Lockhart, 1972). Crystallized intelligence changes very little throughout the adult life span, while fluid intelligence changes dramatically (Horn & Cattell, 1972). In contrast, other investigators concluded that age-related deficits are distributed throughout the information processing system, rather than localized in a particular stage or process (Birren, 1965; Cerella, Poon, & Williams, 1980; Cerella, 1990; Hale, Myerson, & Wagstaff, 1987; Myerson et al., 1990; Salthouse, 1985). The difference could be purely semantic in that one category of investigators focuses on a specific stage or a set of processes, while the other examines larger systems in which differential age-related influences are taken into account. Nevertheless, there are substantial differences in methods of synthesis and approach in these two views.

An example of the systems approach focuses on the robust age-by-task complexity phenomenon reported earlier (e.g., Cerella, Poon, & Williams, 1980). That is, age had little or minimal effect in the ability to perform simple tasks with minimal cognitive load but had significant effect on the ability to perform more complex and demanding tasks with higher cognitive leads. This age-by-task phenomenon exists whether the increased difficulty is in levels of the same task or across tasks that vary in difficulty (McDowd & Craik, 1988). From this perspective, the systems approach samples age-related performances across a diversity of cognitive domains and makes conclusions about the characteristics of the younger and older information processors in meeting the task demands.

This systems approach has been used in identifying the general slowing and relative proficiency of information processing in normal (Cerella, Poon, & Williams, 1980; Cerella, 1990; Hale, Myerson, & Wagstaff, 1987; Myerson et al., 1990) and pathological (Poon, 1993; Nebes, & Madden, 1988) aging. The performance of older adults was found to decline proportionally across a range of tasks and cognitive demands (Cerella, Poon, & Williams, 1980). For example, card sorting exhibited a proportional difference of 8 percent, stimulus-response mapping of 32 percent, memory scanning of 40 percent, and so on. When all the tasks were analyzed collectively, an average decrement of 14 percent was found in sensorimotor tasks, which are tasks that employ minimal cognitive load. An average of 62 percent decrement was found in central processing tasks, which are tasks that require a higher cognitive load.

Poon (1993) administered a battery of cognitive tasks that were found to be sensitive to pathological changes to young, middle-aged, and older adults. He found systematic changes in processing functions as a function of age. He further administered the same battery to patients with early dementia but without depression, those with major depression but with no dementia, and age-matched controls. He found significant decrement patterns for the patients who had early dementia but no major depression.

Taken together, the systems approach was found to be sensitive in mapping and quantifying the integrity of information processors in aging and pathology. Owing to the systematic and generalized nature of cognitive decrement in aging, several postulations have been forwarded, which include the slowing of the central nervous system (Birren, 1965), general resource decrement (Salthouse, 1988, 1997), and decrement in neural network (Cerella, 1990).

Although the fitness–task complexity phenomenon is widely reported in the literature (e.g., Chodzko-Zajko & Moore, 1994), the authors of this chapter were interested in quantifying the relative magnitudes of differences between highly fit and less fit older adults. We reanalyzed data from 10 often-cited studies that reported a positive relationship between fitness and cognitive functions and examined the relative performances, or proportional ratios (H/L), of highly fit (H) versus less fit (L) older adults (see table 3.1). Tasks from the 10 studies were divided into three categories: lower, medium, and higher cognitive demand. Tasks with lower cognitive demand required no or very little processing, such as simple reaction time, digit comprehension, digit span, vocabulary, and tapping. Tasks with higher cognitive demand required the most processing, such as memory retrieval, decision and discrimination, trail making, and sorting tasks. Examples of intermediate demand included making choices, analogies, reading, number span, and comparisons.

The average proportional ratios for low cognitive demands is 1.0 or no difference, 1.12 or 12 percent for medium load, and 1.55 or 55 percent for a high cognitive load. When high cognitive demands are needed, the differences between highly fit and less fit older adults are profound, in the range of 50 to 100 percent. Taken together, the analysis showed that systematic decrement is evident in less fit older adults when compared to highly fit older adults. The finding of generalized decrement in less fit older adults is similar to the functional age model reviewed by Stones and Kozma (1988) (see chapter 2). Therefore, exercise exerts general benefits to the overall health and cognitive functioning of the aging organism.

Is Fitness a Protective Factor Against "Usual" Age-Related Declines in Cognition?

We have reviewed research findings and resulting hypotheses that support the concept that age-related cognitive decrements are most evident in complex tasks with a high cognitive load in which decision-making, attention-demanding, and executive functions are necessary. In our earlier research, we estimated that older adults, compared to younger adults, on average were 60 percent less proficient on complex cognitive tasks (Cerella, Poon, & Williams, 1980). Yet, researchers have also repeatedly shown that fitness reduced cognitive deficits in precisely the same complex central executive function tasks with a high cognitive load. Our estimate from data on highly fit and less fit older adults showed that sedentary older adults could be 55 percent less proficient. From these findings, it seems reasonable to suggest that although aging exerts detrimental effects on many types of cognition, the maintenance of at least moderate levels of physical fitness provides restorative effects. Furthermore, low fitness levels exacerbate age-related declines in cognition, especially processes that are complex. One could therefore postulate that low fitness levels may be viewed as a risk factor for cognitive health, while high fitness levels may provide a protective factor.

Conclusion

The goal of this chapter is to integrate and extend concepts reviewed in chapters 1 and 2. Particularly, extant data that support the conclusion that fitness could facilitate cognitive functions in old age. What is the magnitude of the fitness effect on older adults? The literature is clear

Table 3.1   Summary of 10 Studies

Authors	Study type	Sample	Tasks
Abourezk, T. (1989)	Cross-sectional: No exercise intervention and no random subject assignment	20 male volunteers age 50-70 A) 10 active B) 10 inactive	Heart rate Blood pressure Systolic Diastolic Dichotic listening Digit comprehension Selection Attention Short-term memory 1st ear 2nd ear
Baylor, A.M., & Spirduso, W.W. (1988)	Cross-sectional: No exercise intervention and no random assignment	16 females age 48-63 A) Active B) Inactive	Reaction time Premotor time Movement time Contractile time

	Mean results		Proportional ratio (H/L)
Baseline	Highly fit (H)	Less fit (L)	
Health	Heart rate	Heart rate	
Active: Runs 25 miles	A) 53.20	B) 72.20	1.36 (nr)
per wk	Blood pressure	Blood pressure	
A) Heart rate: 53.2	Systolic	Systolic	
BP: 107-70	A) 107	B) 122	1.14 (nr)
Inactive: Did not do,	Diastolic	Diastolic	
and had never	A) 70	B) 76	1.09 (nr)
participated in,	Dichotic listening	Dichotic listening	
aerobic exercise.	Digit comprehension	Digit comprehension	
B) Heart rate: 72.2	A) 99.70	B) 99.50	1.00 (ns)
BP: 122-76	Selection attention	Selection attention	
Cognition	A) 92.65	B) 91.25	1.02 (ns)
No baseline assess-	Short-term memory	Short-term memory	
ment	1st ear	1st ear	
	A) 23.10	B) 22.20	1.04 (ns)
	2nd ear	2nd ear	
	A) 13.40	B) 6.70	2.00 (0.05)
Health	Reaction time	Reaction time	
No baseline assess-	A) 267	B) 348	1.30 (0.05)
ment	Premotor time	Premotor time	
Cognition	SRT	SRT	
No baseline assess-	A) 164	B) 203	1.24 (ns)
ment	DRT	DRT	
	A) 211	B) 291	1.38 (0.05)
	Movement time	Movement time	
	A) 161	B) 258	1.60 (0.05)
	Contractile time	Contractile time	
	A) 79	B) 101	1.28 (0.05)

(continued)

Table 3.1   *(continued)*

Authors	Study type	Sample	Tasks
Clarkson-Smith, L., & Hartley, A.A. (1989)	Cross-sectional: No exercise intervention and no random assignment	124 male & female volunteers (either high or low exercise) A) High exercise B) Low exercise	Heart rate Blood pressure Systolic Diastolic Reasoning Analogies Matrices Series Working memory Letter sets Reading span Digit span Reaction time Total RT M Total SD M Slope
Dustman, R.E., Emmerson, R.Y., Ruhling, R.O., Shearer, D.E., Steinhaus, L.A., Johnson, S.C., Bonekat, H.W., & Shigeoka, J.W. (1990)	Cross-sectional: Correlational with no exercise intervention and no random assignment	60 males age 20-31, 50-62 A) 15 young highly fit B) 15 young less fit C) 15 old highly fit D) 15 old less fit	$\dot{V}O_2$max Vocabulary Reaction time (Sternberg) Stroop color Symbol digit Trails B (Cognitive measures combined to a composite)

	Mean results		Proportional ratio (H/L)
Baseline	**Highly fit (H)**	**Less fit (L)**	
<u>Health</u>	Heart rate	Heart rate	
High: Self-rated	A) 66.23	B) 70.85	0.93 (0.05)
health (M = 6.03)	Blood pressure	Blood pressure	
Strenuous activity	Systolic	Systolic	
(M = 5.66 h/wk)	A) 131.51	B) 134.23	1.02 (ns)
Low: Self-rated	Diastolic	Diastolic	
health (M = 5.11)	A) 77.72	B) 77.61	1.00 (ns)
Strenuous activity	Reasoning	Reasoning	
(M = 0.01 h/wk)	Analogies	Analogies	
<u>Cognition</u>	A) 23.97	A) 21.29	1.13 (0.001)
High: 16.62 yrs edu-	Matrices	Matrices	
cation	A) 15.55	A) 11.82	1.32 (.001)
Low: 15.37 yrs edu-	Series	Series	
cation	A) 12.08	A) 10.04	1.20 (0.001)
	Working memory	Working memory	
	Letter sets	Letter sets	
	A) 46.42	A) 34.16	1.36 (0.001)
	Reading span	Reading span	
	A) 13.69	A) 10.97	1.25 (0.05)
	Digit span	Digit span	
	A) 26.13	A)26.39	0.99 (ns)
	Reaction time	Reaction time	
	Total RT M	Total RT M	
	A) 514.84	A) 574.34	1.12 (.001)
	Total SD M	Total SD M	
	A) 158.78	A) 187.07	1.18 (.01)
	Slope	Slope	
	A) 2.07	A) 2.48	1.20 (.01)
<u>Health</u>	$\dot{V}O_2$max	VO_2	
$\dot{V}O_2$max	A) 60.5	B) 38.4	1.58 (nr)
Highly fit:	C) 49.8	D) 29.1	1.71 (nr)
A) 60.5	Vocabulary	Vocabulary	
C) 53.8	A) 59.8	B) 61.3	0.98 (ns)
Less fit:	C) 64.7	D) 60.1	1.08 (0.03)
B) 38.4	Cognition	Cognition	
D) 29.1	A) 108	B) 105	1.03 (.02)
<u>Cognition</u>	C) 99	D) 87	1.14 (.02)
Vocabulary			
Highly fit:			
A) 59.8			
C) 64.7			
Less fit:			
B) 61.3			
D) 60.1			

(continued)

Table 3.1   *(continued)*

Authors	Study type	Sample	Tasks
Emmerson, R.Y., Dustman, R.E., & Shearer, D.E. (1990)	Cross-sectional: Correlational with no exercise intervention and no random assignment	60 individuals age 20-31, 50-62 A) 15 young highly fit B) 15 young less fit C) 15 old highly fit D) 15 old less fit (because no age by fitness interactions were significant, the groups were collapsed by fitness level)	Reaction time (Sternberg) Trail-making task Stroop test
Rikli, R., & Busch, S. (1986)	Cross-sectional: Correlational with no exercise intervention and no random assignment	60 females A) 15 young active ($M = 22.2$) B) 15 young inactive ($M = 21.1$) C) 15 older active ($M = 68.7$) D) 15 older inactive ($M = 68.9$)	Reaction time Simple RT Choice RT
Sherwood, D.E., & Selder, D.J. (1979).	Cross-sectional: Correlational with no exercise intervention and no random assignment	64 volunteers age 23-59 A) 33 active (22 M, 10 F) B) 32 inactive (20 M, 12 F)	Reaction time Simple RT Choice RT

| | Mean results | | Proportional ratio |
Baseline	Highly fit (H)	Less fit (L)	(H/L)
Health Active: Inactive: Cognition Active: 138.9 Inactive: 134.25	Reaction time (Sternberg) 138.9 Trail-making task 30.6 Stroop test 7.15	Reaction time (Sternberg) 134.25 Trail-making task 49.5 Stroop test 9.1	0.97 (ns) 1.62 (0.05) 1.27 (0.02)

Health
Active: Vigorous
  activity 3 × wk for 3
  yrs (young) and 10
  yrs (old)
Inactive: No vigorous
  activity on regular
  basis
Cognition
No baseline
	SRT
	A) 242.80
	C) 248.60
	CRT
	A) 275.47
	C) 295.13
		SRT
		B) 257.40
		D) 264.20
		CRT
		B) 295.13
		D) 301.20
			1.06
			1.06
			
			1.07
			1.02
			SRT
			Age effect (0.01)
			Fitness effect (0.001)
			Age X fitness effect
			  (ns)
			CRT
			Age effect (0.001)
			Fitness effect (0.001)
			Age by fitness effect
			  (0.05)

Health
Active: Ran 4-7
  miles/day
Inactive: Sedentary
Cognition
Active: 5.5 years
  education beyond
  high school
Inactive: 4.4 yrs edu-
  cation beyond high
  school
	SRT
	A) 195.5
	CRT
	A) 245
		SRT
		B) 205
		CRT
		B) 276
			1.05 (<0.01)
			
			1.12 (<0.01)

(continued)

Table 3.1   *(continued)*

Authors	Study type	Sample	Tasks
Spirduso, W.W. (1975)	Cross-sectional: Correlational with no exercise intervention and no random assignment	60 males age 20-30, 50-70 A) 15 young active ($M = 23.6$) B) 15 young inactive ($M = 25.4$) C) 15 old active ($M = 57.2$) D) 15 old inactive ($M = 56.3$)	Reaction time Simple RT Discrimination RT Movement time Simple MT Discrimination MT
Spirduso, W.W., MacRae, H.H., MacRae, P.G., Prewitt, J., & Osborne L. (1988)	Cross-sectional: Correlational with no exercise intervention and no random assignment	111 females age 20-29, 50-59, 60-69, & 70-79 A) 10 active 20-29 B) 20 inactive 20-29 C) 18 active 50-59 D) 14 inactive 50-59 E) 16 active 60-69 F) 14 inactive 60-69 G) 10 active 70-79 H) 9 inactive 70-79	Reaction time Simple Discrimination (DRT – SRT) Tapping

	Mean results		Proportional ratio (H/L)
Baseline	**Highly fit (H)**	**Less fit (L)**	
Health	Reaction time	Reaction time	
Active:	Simple RT	Simple RT	
A) Racket games for	A) 243	B) 264	1.09 (ns)
2 to 3 yrs (3 times/	C) 263	D) 327	1.24 (<0.05)
wk)	Discrimination RT	Discrimination RT	
C) Racket games for	A) 287	B) 303	1.06 (ns)
last 30 yrs (3 times/	C) 317	D) 355	1.12 (0.05)
wk)	Movement time	Movement time	
Inactive: Never par-	Simple MT	Simple MT	
ticipated in sports in	A) 137	B) 181	1.32 (0.001)
lifetime	C) 149	D) 250	1.68 (0.001)
Cognition	Discrimination MT	Discrimination MT	
No baseline	A) 159	B) 196	1.23 (0.004)
	C) 172	D) 271	1.58 (0.004)
Health	Reaction time	Reaction time	
Active:	Simple*	Simple*	
Inactive:	A) 225	B) 251	1.12 (0.02)**
Cognition	C) 255	D) 278	1.09 (0.02)**
Active:	E) 271	F) 266	0.98 (0.02)
Inactive:	G) 277	H) 281	1.01 (0.02)
	Discrimination*	Discrimination*	
	A) 279	B) 318	1.14 (.002)**
	C) 325	D) 373	1.15 (.002)**
	E) 238	F) 369	1.55 (.002)**
	G) 386	H) 401	1.04 (.002)**
	(DRT – SRT)	(DRT – SRT)	
	A) 51	B) 78	1.53 (0.04)**
	C) 71	D) 92	1.30 (0.04)**
	E) 62	F) 102	1.65 (0.04)**
	G) 109	H) 121	1.11 (0.04)
	Tapping *	Tapping *	
	A) 77	B) 71	1.08 (0.05)**
	C) 71	D) 69	1.03 (.05)
	E) 68	F) 67	1.01 (0.05)
	G) 64	H) 66	0.97 (0.05)

(continued)

Table 3.1 *(continued)*

Authors	Study type	Sample	Tasks
Spirduso, W.W., & Clifford, P. (1978)	Cross-sectional: Correlational with no exercise intervention and no random assignment	90 males age 20-30 ($M = 22.2$), 60-70 ($M = 64.2$) A) 15 young active racket players B) 15 young active runners C) 15 young inactive D) 15 old active racket players E) 15 old active runners F) 15 old inactive	Reaction time Simple RT Choice RT Movement time Simple MT Choice MT

| | Mean results | | Proportional ratio |
Baseline	Highly fit (H)	Less fit (L)	(H/L)
Health	Reaction time	Reaction time	
Active:	Simple RT	Simple RT	
A) Racket games for	A) 243		1.11
2 to 3 wks (4 times/	B) 236	C) 270	1.14
wk)	D) 259		1.15
B) Runner (for past	E) 267	F) 297	1.11
2 to 3 yrs (3 miles, 4	Choice RT	Choice RT	
times/wk)	A) 306		1.08
D) Racket games for	B) 296	C) 331	1.12
last 20 yrs (4 times/	D) 328		1.16
wk)	E) 348	F) 381	1.09
E) Runner for past	Movement time	Movement time	
20 yrs (3 miles, 4	Simple MT	Simple MT	
times/wk)	A) 134		1.14
Inactive: Never par-	B) 119	C) 153	1.29
ticipated in sports in	D) 328		1.31
lifetime	E) 348	F) 185	1.34
Cognition	Choice MT	Choice MT	
No baseline	A) 156		1.13
	B) 139	C) 177	1.27
	D) 175		1.22
	E) 165	F) 214	1.30
			Simple RT
			Choice RT
			Simple MT
			Choice MT
			Activity Effect (<0.05)
			Age Effect (<0.05)
			Interaction (ns)
			On SRT, CRT, SMT, and CMT, the older sports groups were significantly different than both inactive groups. For SMT & CMT, the running groups were significantly faster than racket sports men. Positive Relationship.

that the magnitude depends on the level of cognitive demand necessary for efficiently executing the task. In navigating everyday situations, there is no difference between highly fit and less fit adults in performing routine and automatic tasks (Poon, Rubin, & Wilson, 1989). However, highly fit adults have the advantage in high-stress and challenging attention-intensive situations such as in driving on metropolitan expressways on which cars are traveling at high speeds and in finding the proper exit in an unfamiliar setting.

In our examination of the aging and fitness literature, those mechanisms that seem to be most affected by aging are also the mechanisms that could differentiate highly fit and less fit older adults. We therefore suggest that fitness could be viewed as a protective factor in the maintenance of cognitive health in old age and in high-stress, attention-demanding situations. Although the extant literature provides compelling evidence that fitness is positively related to cognitive functioning, we are in our infancy in understanding the intervening mechanisms that would enable fitness to facilitate cognition in old age. For example, potential intervening or mediating mechanisms that are particularly germane to exercise and cognition are physical resources (e.g., energy, sleep, appetite,), mental resources (e.g., motivation, stress adaptation, depression), and disease states (e.g., hypertension, diabetes) (Spirduso, Poon, & Chodzko-Zajko, in press). How do these mechanisms independently and collectively affect cognitive performances? Explications of these direct and indirect effects are planned for volume II of this series.

CHAPTER 4

Effect of Exercise on Cognition in Older Adults: A Reexamination of Proposed Mechanisms

Robert E. Dustman, PhD, and Andrea White, PhD

In the mid-1970s, bones of one of our ancient ancestors were found in a remote area of Africa (Johanson & Edey, 1981). An examination of this partial skeleton, named *Lucy,* and the bones of other prehumans of the same species, Australopithicus afarensis, who lived at least 3.5 million years ago indicated that members of this species walked in an upright manner similar to that of people today and were capable of vigorous physical activity (Åstrand, 1992; Park, 1992). It has been suggested that nearly 100 percent of the existence of the hominid/homo species was spent as hunter-gatherers and that today we are genetically adapted to a lifestyle of strenuous outdoor activity (Åstrand, 1988; Åstrand & Rodahl, 1986; Bortz, 1989), adaptations that extend to our emotional and social lives and to our cognitive skills, as well. Cohen (1987) stated that modern man is living in a biological time warp with Stone Age physiologies that are attempting to adapt to modern-day lifestyles that include new diets and too little exercise (Bortz, 1989). A report stated that 75 percent of all deaths in Western nations are the result of lifestyles that deviate substantially from those of our hunter-gatherer ancestors (Eaton, Konner, & Shostak, 1988). The fundamental biological principles for existence we have inherited predated the Australopithicus genus by hundreds of millions of years (Åstrand, 1994; Eaton, Konner, & Shostak, 1988). Because of our genetic background, it should not be surprising that individuals who maintain relatively high levels of physical fitness would enjoy better physical and brain health than those who lead more sedentary lifestyles. Strenuous exercise may be *essential* for optimum functioning.

Rowe and Kahn (1987) differentiate between *usual* and *successful* aging. Lifestyles of individuals who age "successfully" are more likely to include health-promoting practices that contribute to maintenance of physical and behavioral functioning into old age. These health-promoting practices include frequent physical exercise, healthful diets, and activities that improve psychosocial well-being. Of these, physical exercise—particularly aerobic exercise—has been shown to significantly reduce the incidence of several diseases that frequently occur in older adults, for example, cardiovascular disease, stroke, diabetes, colon cancer, and osteoporosis (Rowe & Kahn, 1998). Physical exercise also improves strength, stamina, and vigor, which are important for the maintenance of independence in old age. And, directly contributing to overall health of the central nervous system (CNS) are the beneficial effects that strenuous exercise has on the cardiovascular system.

It is not surprising that exercise-induced improvements in cardiovascular health are paralleled by improvements in CNS health and function because the cardiovascular system transports oxygen and glucose to the brain. Evidence of a link between cardiovascular health and CNS health was reported during the early years of the electroencephalogram (EEG). Investigators found that cardiovascular disease was associated with an increased incidence of EEG abnormalities and decreased cognitive abilities. On the other hand, data from aerobically trained animals and humans have shown a positive relationship between cardiovascular and CNS health. Studies with animals (primarily rats) have documented a direct influence of aerobic exercise on CNS health. Performance of aerobically trained rats on tests of learning and memory is superior to performance of nontrained animals (Fordyce & Farrar, 1991; Fordyce & Wehner, 1993; Spencer, Mattsson, Johnson, & Albee, 1993; Spirduso & Farrar, 1981), and structural, chemical, and vascular changes have been reported to occur in the brains of exercised rats, changes that would be expected to improve CNS efficiency (Black, 1998; DeCastro & Duncan, 1985; Fordyce & Farrar, 1991; Rosenzweig & Bennett, 1996).

Concerning humans, many reports document that older adults who have maintained a relatively high level of aerobic fitness over a substantial period of time have consistently performed better on neuropsychological tests than more sedentary people of similar age. However, findings from longitudinal studies in which older sedentary people have participated in an aerobic exercise program for periods extending over months rather than years have not been as consistent. Although some investigators have reported that aerobic exercise resulted in improved performance on cognitive tests involving "mental flexibility" and speed of responding (Dustman et al., 1984; Hawkins, Kramer, & Capaldi, 1992; Kramer et al., 1999; Moul, Goldman, & Warren, 1995; Spirduso & Farrar, 1981; Stacey, Kozma, & Stones, 1985), others have not found that aerobic exercise facilitates cognitive functioning (Blumenthal & Madden, 1988; Madden, Blumenthal, Allen, & Emery, 1989; Panton et al., 1990). Explanations of the inconsistent results are not readily apparent but may relate to methodological differences among studies in terms of rigor of exercise regimens, subject samples, and other factors (Tomporowski, 1997). Lack of an exercise training effect on cognitive functioning could be caused by an insufficient level of exercise intensity, particularly for older adults who are more likely than young adults to exhibit symptoms of exercise intolerance at high work rates (White et al., 1998). Also, the age at which adults begin a systematic exercise program may be an important factor when evaluating results of human training studies. There is evidence that the older brain loses some of its capacity to undergo neurobiological change (Dustman, Emmerson, & Shearer, 1994). Taken as a whole, however, results from animal intervention studies and human cross-sectional and intervention studies do appear to provide supportive evidence of a connection between aerobic fitness status and neurocognitive function (Dustman et al., 1994).

If strenuous exercise is related to improved brain functioning, what are the intervening mechanisms? One might expect that the mechanisms would be related to basic functional properties of the brain such as cerebral blood flow (CBF), neurotransmitter function, the oxidation of glucose, which provides needed energy for a highly metabolic organ, brain plasticity, and the interplay between CNS excitation and inhibition, which governs all behaviors.

Metabolism

The brain consumes a large amount of energy in the maintenance of physical and mental functioning (Meyer et al., 1976). Although comprising only 2 percent of the total body weight, the brain uses 20 to 25 percent of the total body oxygen and 25 percent of the total body glucose to meet the brain's energy needs and for the metabolism and turnover of neurotransmitters (Friedland, 1990). These facts and the knowledge that the practice of aerobic exercise promotes an increase in the oxygen-carrying capacity of red blood cells and facilitates the transport and delivery of oxygen to working cells has contributed to an expectation that aerobic fitness may be linked to cognitive functioning. McFarland published a paper in 1963, *Experimental Evidence of the Relationship Between Aging and Oxygen Want: In Search of a Theory,* in which he proposed ". . . the aging process concerns the diminished ability of the organism to transport and utilize oxygen in all tissues of the body, and especially in the central nervous system" (p. 341). Supportive evidence for his theory was provided by studies that investigated physiological and cognitive behaviors of young adults who had undergone periods of forced physical deconditioning or who were experiencing hypoxia while at altitude or in a hypobaric chamber. McFarland noted that in a number of respects, physiological and cognitive functioning of hypoxic young adults was similar to that of elderly people. As an example, vision is quite susceptible to oxygen want (McFarland, 1968; Wolf & Nadroskik,

1971) and declines during the process of aging (Weale, 1986). Wolf and Nadroski (1971) reported that a reduction in oxygen tension of inhaled air reduced visual sensitivity of young adults to a level observed for subjects who were 30 to 50 years older; the authors suggested that the visual impairment experienced by the young adults was related to a slowing of retinal metabolism. The retina, a part of the CNS, is known to have a high metabolic rate (Ernest & Krill, 1971).

Findings from two investigations suggest that aerobic fitness is related to visual sensitivity in older adults. Dustman and colleagues reported that a four month–long walking program improved the critical flicker fusion (CFF) threshold of older adults (CFF threshold is the frequency at which a train of flashes is perceived to fuse into a continuous light and is known to be sensitive to hypoxia) (Dustman et al., 1984). A second study (Dustman, Emmerson, Ruhling, Shearer, Steinhaus, Johnson, et al. 1990) demonstrated that both the CFF threshold and visual sensitivity threshold of aerobically fit young and old men were superior to thresholds of age-matched subjects who seldom exercised (visual sensitivity threshold was the lowest illumination at which a visual stimulus could be perceived).

Cerebral Blood Flow

Oxygen and glucose are not stored in the brain; thus the vascular system must quickly respond to environmental demands on the CNS by resupplying activated brain areas with these substances. The vascular system and the CNS work together very well in this regard. The idea that cerebral perfusion is tightly coupled to neuronal activity was advanced more than 100 years ago by Roy & Sherrington (1890). They hypothesized that ". . . . the chemical products of cerebral metabolism contained in the lymph which bathes the walls of the arterioles of the brain can cause variations of the caliber of the cerebral vessels. In this reaction the brain possesses an intrinsic mechanism by which its vascular supply can be varied locally in correspondence with local variations of functional activity" (p. 105). These were astute observations and, with few exceptions, their hypothesis has been well supported.

A number of vasoactive substances have been found that are purported to autoregulate CBF by *constricting* and *dilating* blood vessels. For example, the catecholamines, acetylcholine, some peptides (Lou, Edvinsson, & MacKenzie, 1987) and carbon dioxide (Globus et al., 1983; Ide & Secher, 2000) have been reported to act as autoregulators. Constriction of vessels during relatively high neural activity is important for the prevention of elevated CBF and the accompanying high systolic blood pressure that could damage blood vessels (Carey et al. , 2000). In addition, blood vessel constriction results in faster flow rates to offset the absence of additional CBF during periods of heightened neural activity (Ide & Secher, 2000; Jiang et al., 1995; Jorgensen, Perko, & Secher, 1992).

According to Lou, Edvinsson, and MacKenzie (1987), blood vessels themselves may assist in governing an accurate and speedy delivery of blood to activated brain tissue. The authors emphasize that all parts of the cerebral circulation have a rich perivascular nerve supply that may serve as an alternative control system to allow for rapid and parallel changes in flow and neuronal activity. It has been reported that local blood flow increases can occur as soon as one second after neuronal activation with a spatial distribution restricted to a very small area, about 25 µm (Silver, 1978). Thus, the coupling of CBF to neural activity can be tuned quickly and precisely.

Cerebral Blood Flow and Aging

Most of the reviewed evidence regarding CBF in healthy older adults strongly suggests that age is inversely related to efficient delivery of blood to the CNS (Leenders et al., 1990; Marchal et al., 1992; Slosman et al., 2001; Takada et al., 1992). An age-related reduction in CBF has been estimated to range from 30 to 60 ml per kg of brain per minute per year across studies. It should be noted, however, that the lower figure was from a sample of 187 adults that contained only 3 subjects older than 60 years old. In a study of 27 healthy subjects age 19 to 76 years, Meltzer and colleagues (2000) also reported an age-related drop in CBF. However, after correcting data for brain tissue loss in older subjects, the age difference disappeared, suggesting that tissue *perfusion* may not change with age. If age-related reductions in CBF become excessive, an ischemic threshold can be reached such that a shift to increased anaerobic glycolysis occurs (Meyer, Terayama, & Takashima, 1993).

CBF levels in adult males and females have been reported to differ (Meyer, Terayama, & Takashima, 1993; Slosman et al., 2001): CBF of women is significantly higher that that of men until the age of menopause when male–female differences in CBF become progressively smaller.

The velocity of cerebral blood flow has been reported to slow during adult aging (Ajmani et al., 2000). Ajmani and colleagues investigated age changes in hemorheological properties and CBF velocity in a sample of 147 individuals age 26 to 98 years (rheology is the study of the deformation and flow of matter). Findings from this study indicated several hemorheological age changes that would be expected to interfere with blood transport. These include age-related increases in whole-blood viscosity, plasma viscosity, and aggregation. These alterations in blood flow properties together with age-related changes in cerebrovascular resistance, which reflect loss of elasticity and progressive fibrosis of cerebral vasculature (Meyer, Terayama, & Takashima., 1993), undoubtedly contribute to the slowing of blood flow velocity. In spite of the age losses cited earlier, dynamic cerebral autoregulation, the ability to maintain blood flow changes occurring over a matter of seconds, did not differ between a group of 27 healthy young adults who were less than or equal to 40 years of age and an older group of 27 subjects age 55 years and older (Carey et al., 2000).

A study by Rogers, Meyers, and Mortel (1990) demonstrated that physical activity can help to maintain cerebral perfusion during the aging process. Three groups of 30 postal workers who were of retirement age were enrolled in a four-year prospective longitudinal investigation of relationships between physical activity and cerebral perfusion. One group planned to defer retirement for five years; the remaining 60 individuals planned to retire at the beginning of the study. The latter subjects were assigned to one of two subgroups based on physical activity levels: retired, active and retired, inactive. Mean activity level of the subjects in the retired, inactive group was significantly lower than that of the nonretired and the retired, active groups. Over the four-year experimental period, CBF levels for the retired physically inactive group progressively declined, while CBF levels of the active groups remained relatively stable.

Oxygen Administration and Cognition

Not only is oxygen essential for the complete metabolism of glucose, which maintains brain energy levels but also for the metabolism of some neurotransmitters, notably acetylcholine and the biogenic amines dopamine, norepinephrine, and serotonin (Davis, Carlsson, MacMillan, & Siesjo, 1973; Davis, Giron, Stanton, & Maury, 1979; Gibson & Peterson, 1982). In vitro studies indicated that alterations in oxygen levels of room air resulted in parallel changes in neurotransmitter function. Endurance exercise training of rodents, which increases oxygen transport and delivery to cerebral tissue, also has been demonstrated to improve functioning of acetylcholine and the biogenic amines (Brown & Van Huss, 1973; DeCastro & Duncan, 1985; Gilliam et al., 1984; Samorajski, Rolsten, Przykorska, & Davis, 1987). Although not proven, the exercise-related changes in neurotransmitter activity may well be related to increased oxygenation of brain stem neuronal sites specific to the above transmitters.

During the past few years, a small group of investigators in the United Kingdom has been engaged in unraveling relationships between cerebral oxygenation and cognition in a fairly straightforward manner. Although the studies have been conducted with college-age students, their procedures and results would appear to have relevance to future metabolic studies of aging. For this reason four of their published papers on oxygen and cognition are briefly described.

The first study (Moss & Scholey, 1996), composed of three experiments, was designed to evaluate the effects of oxygen inhalation on memory. One hundred and five young adults were randomly assigned to one of three groups: (a) inhale pure oxygen through a face mask for 60 seconds immediately prior to a visual administration of a 15-item word list, (b) inhale oxygen immediately prior to a recall test that occurred 10 minutes following word presentation, and (c) control (no intervention). The investigators found that oxygen inhalation had a beneficial effect on memory consolidation but not on memory retrieval. Subjects who were administered oxygen immediately *before* word list presentation recalled a significantly larger number of words than subjects in the control group and in the experimental group who received oxygen at the time of word retrieval.

A second experiment extended the time between word list exposure and word list retrieval to 24 hours but with other experimental parameters left unchanged. Again, compared to the two comparison groups, delayed recall was significantly better for those individuals who inhaled oxygen at the time of word list presentation.

To rule out effects related to subjects' expectations that oxygen should improve memory, a third experiment was conducted. In this experiment, one group of 12 subjects inhaled oxygen while an equal number of subjects inhaled air; procedures ensured that subjects were blind regarding the gas being administered. The interval between list learning and memory retrieval was again 24 hours. Results from this experiment eliminated expectation as a possible explanation of their earlier findings because the number of words recalled by subjects receiving oxygen was reliably larger than the number recalled by the individuals who breathed air.

A second study utilized a more complex experimental design to examine the effects of oxygen inhalation on cognitive performance (Moss, Scholey, & Wesnes, 1998). Ten cognitive tests, each part of a computerized cognitive assessment battery, were administered. The test variables were grouped into three categories: attention, long-term memory, and working memory. Computer programs controlled test administration and scoring as well as the delivery of oxygen and air to a face mask from compressed air cylinders through quick-release valves.

Each of 20 trained subjects (21-48 yrs, mean = 24.5) participated in five randomly ordered experimental conditions: continuous air throughout the testing session (control), continuous oxygen during the session, 30 seconds of oxygen prior to each task in the battery, and 1 or 3 minutes of oxygen prior to the session.

Cognitive performance was enhanced by the inhalation of oxygen for some tasks but not for others. For example, oxygen speeded performance on simple and complex reaction time tests and enhanced scores on tests of number vigilance and immediate and delayed word recall but did not improve working and spatial memory. In general, the conditions that were most effective for improving cognitive performance were the administration of 30 seconds of oxygen immediately before individual tests and one and three minutes of oxygen inhalation just prior to test battery administration. Breathing oxygen throughout the test session had little effect on performance. The authors had no explanation for the weaker effects of continuous oxygen on test performance relative to transient infusions of the gas.

A third study investigated temporal relationships between hyperoxia and enhanced memory (Scholey, Moss, & Wesnes, 1998). Twenty young adults participated in experimental conditions that included inhaling air throughout testing (control), receiving 2 minutes of oxygen either 10 minutes, 5 minutes, or immediately before visual presentation of a word list, immediately after the word list, and at the end of a 12-minute test battery that ended with word recall. The test battery also included the digit span tests. The study protocol, including the delivery of air and oxygen, was similar to that reported by Moss and colleagues (1998) with the exception that oxygen hemoglobin saturation was measured at intervals throughout the experiment.

Two findings were of note. (1) Compared to air, oxygen again had a significant effect on word recall. Oxygen selectively enhanced word recall when delivered 5 minutes prior to and immediately before and after word list presentation. Administering oxygen 10 minutes prior to or 5 minutes and 10 minutes after word list presentation did not enhance memory. Oxygen had no effect on digit span. (2) The profile of hemoglobin saturation closely paralleled word recall results: hyperoxia was evident immediately prior to, during, or immediately following word list presentation at the times when word recall was enhanced.

In a continuation of this series of studies, 32 young adults were randomly assigned to air inhalation or oxygen inhalation groups in an investigation of cognitive performance, hyperoxia, and heart rate (Scholey, Moss, Neave, & Wesnes, 1999). Cognition was assessed by a memory test (word recall) and a reaction time test; the tests were from the computerized test battery. Gas delivery procedures were similar to those in the previous two studies. Oxygen or air was delivered for 70 seconds just prior to the time subjects were presented with a word list. A test of word recall occurred 5.5 minutes later. Blood oxygen saturation level and heart rate were measured at regular intervals throughout the experiment.

As expected, cognitive performance was enhanced by the administration of oxygen. A questionnaire asking subjects which gas they received indicated that subjects did not recognize the difference between pure oxygen and air. For the oxygen-treated group there was a significant negative relationship between *baseline* oxygen saturation level and the number of words recalled. On the basis of these results, the authors suggested that the cognitive-enhancing effect of oxygen may be more pronounced when there is a greater potential for increasing blood oxygen saturation levels. The investigators also reported that heart rates were elevated during the performance of cognitive tests under both the oxygen and air administration conditions. Faster heart rates would be expected to benefit activated neural tissue by providing more frequent deliveries of oxygen and glucose.

Results from these studies seem even more impressive given the age of their subjects, predominantly young adults, at an age when body and brain functioning is at a high level and coincident with relatively high levels of blood oxygen saturation. This and the finding that cognitive functioning of young adults who had the lowest blood saturation levels demonstrated the largest improvements in cognitive functioning suggest that the procedures employed in these studies should be most useful in investigations of oxygen–cognition relationships in older adults who would be expected to be mildly hypoxic.

Glucose Administration and Cognition

The role of glucose in neurocognitive functioning has been studied for many years based on the observations that decreased levels of blood glucose have been shown to impair cognitive function (Frier, 2001; Hall & Gold, 1986; McAulay, Deary, Ferguson, & Frier, 2001) and that glucose supplementation appears to improve cognitive function (Gold, 1995; Hall & Gold, 1986; Scholey, Harper, & Kennedy, 2001; Wenk, 1989). There are several proposed mechanisms that have been suggested to explain these beneficial effects of glucose (Wenk, 1989). Perhaps the most obvious of these is the role of glucose as an energy source for brain activity. More energy availability should lead to enhanced brain functioning.

A review of recent articles regarding the role of glucose in human cognition, and particularly for memory, follows. The interpretation of this research is complicated by the employment of differing concentrations and timing of glucose doses and the relative effectiveness of placebos to mimic glucose in taste. Further, discrepancies between blood glucose values and actual levels in the brain have not been measured in humans. Finally, glucose administrations produce variable results according to the level of cognitive demand and cognitive domain assessed.

The first reviewed study (Winder & Borrill, 1998) bridges the gap between oxygen and glucose administration and was designed to determine the effectiveness of oxygen, glucose, or a combination of oxygen and glucose on memory enhancement. One hundred and four adults whose ages ranged from 18 to 55 years (mn = 29) were randomly assigned to one of four conditions: pure oxygen with a placebo drink, pure oxygen with glucose, air with glucose, and air with a placebo drink. Oxygen and air were delivered from compressed air tanks to a face mask; subjects were blinded with regard to air and drink conditions. Two memory tasks that mimicked tasks carried out in everyday life were administered 15 minutes after an experimental treatment. Subjects were shown a display of 12 photographs of faces with names (name and face association) and a 12-item grocery list (selective reminding test). Subjects were tested on each memory task following a brief distracting task (short-term memory) and again 8 minutes later (long-term memory).

Inhalation of oxygen had a beneficial effect on long-term memory but not on short-term memory, and a combination of oxygen and glucose resulted in memory scores being slightly better than scores for oxygen alone. Surprisingly, the glucose and air condition had no effect on either long-term or short-term memory despite other reports of memory enhancement following glucose administration (see studies cited later) and the fact that the glucose dose used in this study was similar to doses that had been effective in other investigations of memory. According to the authors, it is possible that the memory tasks may not have been sufficiently demanding to reveal an effect.

Kennedy and Scholey (2000) investigated the role of physiological arousal in combination with glucose administration on the performance of cognitive tasks of varying difficulty. The authors postulated that accelerated heart rate caused by cognitive demand may be a mechanism for providing additional and needed glucose to activated neural areas.

Twenty young adults were randomly assigned to a glucose or a placebo drink group and participated in two experimental sessions separated by 24 hours with drinks being reversed for the second session. Three 2-minute cognitive tasks—serial 7s, serial 3s, and word retrieval (generating words beginning with an assigned letter)—and a control task (counting to the beat of a metronome) were performed 20 minutes after a glucose or placebo drink. The serial 7s task required subjects to subtract the number seven from a designated start number between 900 and 1,000. The serial 3s task was identical except that it involved subtractions of the number three. The subjects rated the serial 7s task as being the most difficult, followed by word retrieval, and serial 3s as the easiest.

Performance on serial 7s was significantly enhanced by glucose, and a strong trend of better performance was found for word retrieval, but not for serial 3s. Heart rate was related to cognitive performance in three ways: heart rate was highest for the more difficult tasks, subjects with the lowest baseline heart rate performed better on serial 7s, and subjects with low heart rates demonstrated a larger proportional increase in heart rate during periods of cognitive demand.

These data support the notion that glucose administration has a greater effect on cognition when cognitive loads are high, rather than low, as suggested by Winder and Borrill (1998). The findings that individuals who have low baseline heart rates demonstrate a greater responsivity of heart rate to cognitive challenge are intriguing. Aerobic fitness is associated with lower heart rates at rest and with broader ranges of heart rate frequency during physical exercise. Information regarding fitness levels and the exercise histories of subjects in these kinds of studies could be useful when interpreting relationships among cognitive, physiological, and metabolic variables.

Scholey, Harper, and Kennedy (2001) also examined relationships between glucose ingestion and task difficulty. An additional interest was to compare the relationship between the change in glucose levels during a task with a high cognitive load and a somatic control task. The investigators randomly assigned 20 young adults to one of two similarly tasting drink conditions, glucose (25 g) or placebo (30 g of saccharin). Two experimental sessions, separated by a week, were employed; during the second session subjects switched drinks. Over the course of the experiment each subject was tested after imbibing both the glucose and placebo drinks and after participating in four cognitive tasks of varying cognitive demand: serial 7s (high cognitive demand), word retrieval, a test of verbal fluency, and word memory (the word retrieval and word memory tasks were altered to minimize cognitive load). Also, a simple motor task, computer key pressing, was employed. This task was a "somatically matched" control for the serial 7s task, i.e., the task required a similar number of key presses but imposed low cognitive demand. Testing occurred approximately one hour following drink ingestion. Frequent measures of blood glucose levels were obtained to enable the investigators to interpret relationships between changes in blood glucose level and cognitive and control test performance.

As hypothesized, glucose enhanced performance on the cognitively demanding serial 7s test. Glucose drink ingestion had no significant effect on the verbal fluency and word memory tasks, even though glucose had been positively related to these tasks in previous studies. According to the authors, the absence of improvements on these tasks was probably due to their light cognitive loads. Two findings were reported regarding changes in blood glucose levels during test administration: (1) There was a significantly larger fall in blood glucose level during the serial 7s task compared to the key-press control task of the same duration, and (2) the fall in blood glucose was significantly greater following the glucose drink compared to the placebo for both the serial 7s and key-press control tasks.

The study by Scholey and colleagues (2001) supports previous findings of positive relationships between glucose administration and cognitive function and also provides additional evidence that glucose is more likely to benefit performance on difficult than on easy tasks. In addition, the experiment importantly demonstrated that high cognitive loads are associated with a significantly greater uptake of glucose compared to easier task conditions. Although it may seem obvious that reductions in blood glucose level during serial 7s were related to cerebral glucose uptake, the authors emphasize that increased cardiac activity, which occurs during more difficult cognitive tests as well as other test-related physiological indices of arousal, would likely be responsible for a portion of the drop in peripherally measured glucose.

Glucose Administration, Aging, and Cognition

Hall, Gonder-Frederick, Chewning, Silveira, and Gold (1989) investigated the effects of glucose on memory of 12 students age 18 to 23 years and 11 adults age 58 to 77 years (*mn* = 67.4). Experimental procedures encompassed three days. On day one, subjects performed a control task (count backward from the number 20) then, after ingesting either a glucose or placebo drink, they were administered a battery of tests modified from the Wechsler Memory Scale. The tests given in the following order were paired associates, logical memory (presentation of a taped narrative passage with a 15-minute delayed recall), digit span, and visual memory.

On day two, subjects were tested for a 24-hour recall of paired associates, and then they ingested the "other" drink before repeating the battery of memory tests. On the third day, subjects were tested for recall of the paired associates administered the previous day.

Analyses of data revealed that for young and old subjects combined, glucose resulted in memory enhancement for all of the subtests. However, the older individuals fared better than the young adults in this regard. For the older subjects, significant improvements were found for logical memory and for a composite score of all subtests combined; the only memory improvement for the younger subjects was for digit span forward.

Hall and colleagues (1989) also examined relationships between memory and changes in blood glucose levels that occurred during an experiment and found that increases in blood glucose levels associated with memory task performance inversely predicted composite scores of the older, but not the younger, adults. That is, memory performance was poorest in the elderly subjects with the highest peak glucose increases. This subgroup also demonstrated poorer memory during the placebo condition. The authors suggest that impaired glucose tolerance, manifested as an abnormal increase in blood glucose following glucose ingestion, is associated with poor memory but might represent a compensatory mechanism that attenuates the deficit in blood glucose utilization that occurs with age. These data supported previous observations in animals indicating that the dose response curve for the effects of glucose on memory follows an inverted U-shaped curve (Hall & Gold, 1986).

Manning, Parsons, and Gold (1992) administered glucose and placebo drinks to 22 older adults age 60 to 81 years (*mn* = 67) immediately before or after the subjects had been presented with a narrative prose passage. Subjects were immediately tested for recall and tested again 24 hours later.

Regardless of whether the experimental drinks were administered prior to or after exposure to the narrative passage, memory improvement associated with glucose was significantly better than that for the placebo drink.

Relative to memory scores for the placebo drink condition, subjects recalled 53 percent and 62 percent more information, respectively, when glucose was presented before and after the learning phase of the experiment. The importance of the authors' findings relates to the fact that glucose can enhance both memory storage and retrieval in older adults and that the effects of glucose endure over a period of at least 24 hours, indicating that memory enhancement is not just a matter of high glucose levels at the time of retrieval.

A more recent investigation of glucose–memory interactions in older adults, age 60 to 83 years (mean = 67), was conducted by Manning, Stone, Korol, and Gold (1998). A major purpose of the study was to evaluate the effects of glucose on retrieval of narrative material to which subjects were exposed 24 hours previously; glucose was administered just prior to recall (preretrieval). In another phase of the study the authors examined 24-hour recall of similar material, but in this instance glucose was administered just prior to subjects' exposure to the material to be learned (preacquisition). Similar procedures were employed with a placebo drink being substituted for glucose.

Twenty four–hour memory performance associated with glucose administration was found to be substantially better than that for the placebo condition for both the preacquisition and the preretrieval stages, although 24-hour recall scores were reliably higher for the preacquisition compared to the preretrieval stage. The authors stated that this experiment provided the first human evidence that glucose enhances both memory storage and retrieval.

Glucose, Neuroendocrine Function, and Behavior

Many drugs have been tested to determine their ability to enhance learning and memory (Wenk, 1989). Several of these drugs act on the adrenal glands, causing release of epinephrine. Epinephrine release, through a series of steps, leads to increased blood glucose levels, which can significantly affect cholinergic function in the brain. Increased brain glucose levels decrease activity of noradrenergic neurons in the locus coeruleus (Wenk, 1989), a brain area known to inhibit acetylcholine (ACh) availability, by decreasing the activity of an ACh inhibitor. Glucose also functions as a substrate for acetyl CoA (coenzyme A) synthesis, a precursor of ACh; increased ACh availability is hypothesized to positively affect neurocognitive function, particularly learning and memory (Messier, Durkin, Mrabet, & Destrade, 1990; Wenk, 1989).

Epinephrine may directly influence brain function (Wenk, 1989) by increasing neurotransmitter availability, specifically ACh and gamma-aminobutyric acid (GABA). Support for this hypothesis has been demonstrated in studies of adrenalectomized animals (Mondadori & Petschke, 1987) in which cognition-enhancing agents lost their effectiveness.

Epinephrine may be involved in the formation of new memories (Gold, 1995). This has been shown indirectly in animal studies in which the strongest aversive stimulus was associated with the fastest learning, suggesting that hormonal responses to the aversive stimulus were involved. More direct evidence in which epinephrine levels were manipulated via injection also demonstrated that an optimal level of epinephrine produces the greatest learning effects (Gold, 1995).

The work of Kennedy and Scholey (2000) showed that following glucose ingestion, larger increases in heart rates were associated with greater improvements in neurocognition. It is possible that increased epinephrine release, associated with arousal, could have directly or indirectly influenced these results.

It is well documented that epinephrine levels increase during exercise, especially at the onset of exercise (McArdle, Katch, & Katch, 1996). The role that epinephrine plays in mobilizing glucose and enhancing neurotransmitter availability may at least partially explain why increased fitness is associated with better neurocognitive function. It may be that regular, acute bouts of exercise enhance this effect. Vissing, Andersen, and Diemer (1996) have shown that in the rat, exercise significantly increased total glucose utilization by 38 percent.

Messier, Durkin, Mrabet, and Destrade (1990) studied the effects of glucose injections on high-affinity choline uptake in the hippocampus in an experiment designed to simulate a high central demand for ACh by subjecting rats to mental training or to scopolamine. Choline uptake was used as an indirect measure of ACh resynthesis. Results showed significantly increased choline uptake in rats injected with 3 g/kg of glucose after mental training compared to no training. Mentally trained rats had significantly higher choline uptake when injected with saline compared to glucose. A second experiment that utilized injections of scopolamine (a cholinergic agonist) in combination with either saline or glucose showed that choline uptake was less for rats receiving glucose, despite the fact that glucose restored memory. The authors suggested that the results from the two studies may demonstrate that glucose, under conditions of increased neuronal demand for ACh, may facilitate ACh synthesis (Messier et al., 1990).

It has been suggested that decreases in cognitive function with aging may be partially due to the degeneration of central cholinergic systems (Sternberg, Martinez, Gold, & McGaugh, 1985). Evidence suggests that decreased levels of peripheral epinephrine are related to age-related memory deficits (Sternberg et al., 1985). In a study of young (4 mo) and old (24 mo) mice and rats trained in an avoidance task, the older animals demonstrated poor retention compared to the young animals. When 0.01 mg/kg of epinephrine was injected into the animals, memory in both old and young animals improved. The effect was even more pronounced when 0.1 mg/kg of epinephrine was used. These results suggest that memory deficits in aged rodents may be partially caused by decreased central noradrenergic function (Sternberg et al., 1985). Whether certain types of physical activity can effectively activate central noradrenergic function in older humans should be investigated.

Cortical Inhibition and Behavior

All behavior, from the simplest to the most complex, is modulated by the interplay of neuronal excitation and inhibition. The brain, composed of an estimated 50 billion neurons (Bloom, Lazerson, & Hofstadter, 1985), communicates with its external and internal environment by means of waves of neuronal membrane hyperpolarization and depolarization. At neuronal junctions, depolarization triggers the release of neurotransmitters that drift across the synaptic cleft and attach to postsynaptic receptor sites. The transmitters exert one of two effects on postsynaptic membranes: *excitation,* which lowers cell membrane threshold and increases the probability of cell firing, or *inhibition,* which raises membrane thresholds and decreases the probability of cell firing (Dustman, Emmerson, & Shearer, 1990). Thus, the probability of a neuron firing depends on the spatial and temporal summation of these competing electrical inputs. The importance of inhibition was stated by McGeer, Eccles, and McGeer (1978, p. 133): "We can think that inhibition is a sculpturing process. The inhibition, as it were, chisels away at the diffuse and rather amorphous mass of excitatory action and gives a more specific form to the neuronal performance at every stage of synaptic delay."

There is substantial evidence that inhibition strengthens during childhood and adolescence (Dempster, 1992; Harnishfeger & Pope, 1996; Roberts, 1972) and weakens during adult aging (Dywan & Murphy, 1996; McDowd & Filion, 1992; McDowd & Oseas-Kreger, 1991). There is also some evidence to suggest that the practice of physical activity helps to maintain inhibitory strength in old age.

Electrophysiological Evidence of Age Changes in Inhibitory Strength

Electrical activity within and between the central and peripheral nervous systems is a basic substrate of all behavior. Thus, one might expect that age-related deficits in inhibition would be reflected in measures of brain electrical activity.

Perception of Patterned and Unpatterned Flashes

Event-related potentials (ERPs) are small electrical potentials that are elicited by sensory stimuli such as flashes of light, tones or clicks, and shocks to the skin and signal the arrival and perception of stimuli at the cortex. ERP responses to individual stimuli are quite small relative to the background EEG within which they are embedded. However, after a number of individual responses are summed and averaged using computer procedures, the averaged ERP emerges as a stable pattern of positive and negative potentials that span several hundred milliseconds.

One type of ERP is the visually evoked potential (VEP). The configuration of VEPs elicited by patterned flashes (e.g., a checkerboard pattern) is qualitatively and quantitatively different from VEPs elicited by *unpatterned* flashes of light (Beck, 1975; Regan, 1972). It is not surprising that the two kinds of VEPs differ as the visual system is organized to maximize the detection of lines, edges, and contours; inhibition within the retina and visual cortex plays an essential role in the detection of these pattern elements (Hubel, 1988; Hubel & Wiesel, 1962).

To test the hypothesis that inhibitory strength changes across the life span, Dustman, Snyder, and Schlehuber (1981) investigated similarities of "patterned" and "unpatterned" VEPs to determine whether waveforms of the two types of VEPs would be more alike for individuals presumed to have weakened inhibition, children and the elderly, and thus less able to perceive pattern elements than for subjects of intermediate ages with stronger inhibitory systems. Flash intensities were based on individually determined visual thresholds. VEP waveform similarity was determined by correlating the digital values comprising the first 300 milliseconds of a patterned VEP with corresponding digital values of an unpatterned VEP. It was hypothesized that relatively high positive correlations would reflect a higher degree of waveform similarity because of relatively weak visual inhibition, while low correlations would reflect reduced VEP similarity and stronger visual inhibition. Coefficients of correlations were computed for VEPs recorded from 220 healthy males age 4 to 90 years.

As shown in figure 4.1, the top graph of mean correlations of VEPs recorded from occipital scalp (an area overlying primary visual cortex) clearly supported the age-inhibition hypothesis. Similarity of "patterned" versus "unpatterned" VEPs approximated a U-shaped curve across the life span. As smaller correlations reflect a better differentiation of patterned stimuli, the curve suggests that inhibition within the visual system strengthens during childhood development and weakens during adult aging, beginning in the fifth decade. The fact that inhibitory strength did not continue to decline for the oldest group of subjects (71-90 yrs) was believed to reflect a survivor effect, i.e., physiologies of people who live that

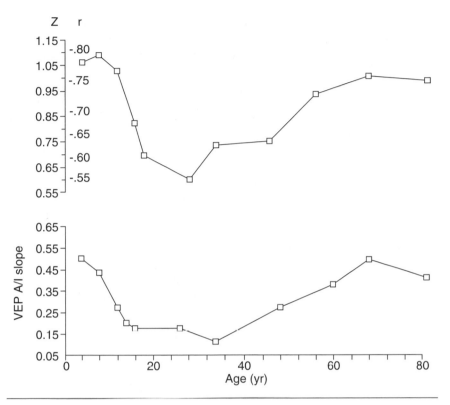

Figure 4.1 Top: Life span changes in similarity of visually evoked potential (VEP) waveforms from occipital scalp that were elicited by patterned and unpatterned flashes. Similarity was determined by correlating digital values of the two types of VEP waveforms. Statistical analyses were done on Fisher Z transformations of coefficients of correlations. Bottom: Mean amplitude-intensity (A/I) slope for 11 groups of 20 males. A/I values were obtained from VEPs recorded at central scalp. Note that both curves support the hypothesis that inhibition strengthens during childhood development and weakens during adult aging.

Reprinted from *Neurobiology of Aging*, R.E. Dustman, E.W. Snyder, and C.J. Schlehuber, Life-span alterna-tions in visually evoked potentials and inhibitory function, pgs. 187-192. Copyright 1981, with permission from Elsevier.

long are probably unusually robust. It should be noted that VEPs recorded from central and frontal scalp areas did not reflect the age changes found at the occipital scalp.

Augmenting and Reducing Visually Evoked Potentials

As flash intensity is increased, VEP amplitude generally increases, although there is considerable variation in the amount of amplitude change among people. It has been theorized that central inhibition governs the relationship between flash intensity and VEP amplitude. The slope of the amplitude-intensity function is presumed to be larger for individuals with weak inhibition because they are less able to dampen their cortical responses to strong flashes while the amplitude-intensity (A/I) slope is of smaller magnitude for individuals with strong inhibition. Thus, we predicted that A/I slope values would be larger for young and old people than for those of intermediate age (Dustman & Snyder, 1981). A/I slope values were computed from VEPs that were recorded from the 220 subjects described in the study just discussed; three flash intensities were employed to elicit VEPs. Inspection of the bottom figure in figure 4.1 shows that the results from this study of inhibition were quite similar to those illustrated in the top figure in figure 4.1. A later investigation studied the effects of aerobic fitness on A/I slope of young and older adults. Each age group was evenly divided between subjects with high and with low $\dot{V}O_2$max values for their age. These data demonstrated that VEP A/I slope values of older men who engaged in aerobic fitness activities on a regular basis were significantly smaller than values for age-matched sedentary men (Dustman, Emmerson, Ruhling, Shearer, et al., 1990) and suggest that the loss of inhibitory strength that occurs in older adults can be slowed by the continued practice of vigorous exercise.

Epilepsy and Seizure Activity

Epilepsy is a disease resulting from a chronic loss of normal balance between excitation and inhibition at synaptic junctions caused by heightened excitability, inhibitory loss, or both (Barlow, 1993; Niedermeyer, 1987). A few studies have been conducted to determine if the practice of physical activity would have an ameliorative effect on the disease, particularly with regards to seizure frequency, which is a reflection of the electrical imbalance.

A 15-week exercise program was conducted with 15 women who had intractable epilepsy (Eriksen et al., 1994). Exercise consisted of aerobic dancing, strength training, and stretching. At the conclusion of the study, mean $\dot{V}O_2$max had increased by 8 percent and plasma cholesterol was decreased, indicating the patients had experienced an aerobic training effect. Patients reported a significant reduction in seizure frequency that endured for a period of three months after cessation of the exercise intervention. During another study, 21 adults with uncontrolled epilepsy participated in a strenuous physical exercise program for a shorter period of time, four weeks (Nakken et al., 1990). Mean $\dot{V}O_2$max increased by 19 percent over the four-week period, and beneficial psychological and social effects were reported. For the group as a whole, however, the exercise intervention did not significantly reduce frequency of seizures, although exercise was related to a reduction in seizure rates for some patients. The authors suggested that enhanced inhibition may be one of the basic mechanisms by which exercise improves seizure control.

Questionnaire data were obtained from a sample of 66 patients with seizures; 36 reported no regular exercise, while 30 had been participating in regular exercise (Denio, Drake, & Pakalnis, 1989). A statistical analysis of these data revealed that patients who regularly exercised had significantly fewer seizures than those who exercised less frequently. Similar findings were obtained from a survey of 204 adult patients with epilepsy (Nakken, 1999). Of those patients, 36 percent reported that regular exercise contributed to better seizure control; 10 percent indicated that exercise tended to precipitate seizures.

Research on rodents has also shown that exercise can have a modulating effect on CNS excitability. Animals that were aerobically trained on running wheels, compared to sedentary animals, produced less spontaneous EEG paroxysmal, seizurelike activity and demonstrated a lower level of CNS sensitivity to behavioral stimulation (Nikiforova, Patchev, & Nikolov, 1989; Nikiforova, Patchev, Nikolov, & Cheresharov, 1988). Finally, aerobic fitness training was shown to be effective in controlling frequency of seizures in rats that had experimentally induced epilepsy (Arida et al., 1999). The positive effect of exercise on seizures extended over a period of 45 days following cessation of the exercise component of the experiment.

It has been suggested that an exercise-induced shift of metabolism toward acidosis increases the level of GABA (Göetze, Kubicki, Munter, & Teichmann, 1967; Nakken et al., 1990). GABA is recognized as being a widespread and important inhibitory neurotransmitter (Roberts, 1972). Thus, increased presence of GABA in the nervous system caused by physical activity may play an important part in maintaining the functional balance between CNS excitation and inhibition.

Although literature regarding relationships between physical exercise and CNS excitatory–inhibitory balance does support the hypothesis that exercise is associated with a strengthening of inhibition within the CNS, the amount of literature that directly focuses on relationships between exercise and excitation and inhibition is quite limited. The importance of further research seems evident particularly for the field of aging; the interaction of excitation and inhibition underlies all behavior, and an increasing imbalance between the two forces has been postulated to occur during adult aging.

Cognitive Evidence of Age Changes in Inhibitory Strength

A sizable body of literature exists concerning tests of hypotheses that age-related weakening of inhibitory strength contributes to cognitive and memory deficits in older adults. This literature is not reviewed here because we are unaware of research studies in which measures of both physical fitness and inhibition have been employed as variables in studies of memory and cognition. Such studies should be fruitful because individual differences in physical fitness might be important in explaining conflicting findings regarding the relationship of inhibition to cognitive functioning.

Exercise and Brain Plasticity

The improved efficiency of cerebral metabolism gained through exercise training enhances brain function. Several studies have demonstrated improved mental function under conditions that supplied more oxygen or glucose or both to the brain (Manning et al., 1998; Moss et al., 1998; Scholey et al., 2001; Scholey et al., 1999) as discussed in previous sections. It has also been determined that voluntary exercise has a direct impact on brain gene expression and thus could be a simple means to maintain brain function and promote brain plasticity (Cotman & Engesser-Cesar, 2002).

A recent, but growing body of research using an animal model has indicated that physical exercise induces a brain-derived neurotrophic factor (BDNF) and other growth factors consistent with improved neuronal activity, synaptic structure, and neuronal plasticity (Cotman & Engesser-Cesar, 2002; Neeper, Gomez-Pinilla, Chol, & Cotman, 1995; Oliff, Berchtold, Isackson, & Cotman, 1998; Tong et al., 2001). BDNF supports the health and functioning of glutaminergic neurons in the brain and stimulates neurogenesis, increases resistance to brain insult, and improves learning and mental function (Cotman & Berchtold, 2002). In exercised rats compared to sedentary rats, increased levels of BDNF have been observed in the hippocampus, an area of the brain important in learning and memory (Cotman & Engesser-Cesar, 2002; Neeper et al., 1995; Oliff et al., 1998; Tong et al., 2001).

Evidence suggests that exercise mediates brain changes acutely. Early studies found a significantly greater abundance of BDNF mRNA (messenger ribonucleic acid) in rat hippocampus, compared to control levels, just six hours after exercise (Oliff et al., 1998). Similarly, BDNF mRNA levels had increased significantly after two to seven days of running (Neeper et al., 1995). A significant, positive correlation was found between mean distance run and BDNF mRNA in the hippocampus (Neeper et al., 1995; Oliff et al., 1998). Additional evidence shows that BDNF action is still observed after six weeks of voluntary wheel running, indicating that the effects are not merely transient responses to acute exercise (Cotman & Engesser-Cesar, 2002).

Further support for the use of exercise as a potential enhancer of mental performance was reported (Russo-Neustadt, Beard, & Cotman,

1999). Because physical activity and antidepressants are often used in the management of Alzheimer's disease, the investigators explored whether either or both of these treatments altered BDNF mRNA expression. Their results indicated that when physical activity (voluntary running by rats) was combined with antidepressant therapy, BDNF mRNA expression in several areas of the hippocampus was increased significantly more than for either treatment alone (Russo-Neustadt et al., 1999). The effect of exercise as an enhancer of this response in humans warrants further investigation.

In the brain, estrogen depletion is associated with decreased BDNF in the hippocampus and decreased neuronal function, survival, and synaptogenesis (Cotman & Engesser-Cesar, 2002). The interaction between exercise and estrogen levels in female rats was recently investigated (Berchtold et al., 2001). To determine how estrogen depletion and exercise might interact to affect BDNF mRNA levels, exercised and sedentary female rats were ovariectomized. It was found that estrogen depletion resulted in significantly decreased activity levels in exercising rats and that estrogen replacement restored previous activity levels. In sedentary animals estrogen depletion reduced baseline BDNF mRNA levels, which were restored with estrogen replacement. With short-term estrogen depletion (3 wks), exercise increased BDNF mRNA levels in areas of the hippocampus. Exercise did not increase BDNF mRNA levels following long-term estrogen depletion (7 wks). Of particular interest was the observation that estrogen combined with exercise increased BDNF mRNA values above the value achieved by estrogen alone. This study appears to have relevance for minimizing the cognitive decline associated with menopause in women as they age; hormone replacement may increase exercise participation and thus induce higher levels of BDNF (Cotman & Engesser-Cesar, 2002). These studies require further investigation in humans.

A recent report by Kramer, Beatty, Plowey, and Waldrop (2002) suggests that exercise may have a much broader effect on brain plasticity than discussed earlier. The investigators studied the effects of exercise on spontaneously hypertensive rats (SHR). It is believed that this type of hypertension is caused by reduced GABAergic influence on regions in the posterior hypothalamus. Because GABAergic activity inhibits tonic excitatory cardiovascular outflow, reductions in GABA influence result in increases in blood pressure (Kramer, Beatty, Plowey, & Waldrop, 2002). Studies of SHR have demonstrated a direct relationship between the intensity of muscle contraction and neuronal firing rate in the posterior hypothalamus. Further, the authors demonstrated that 10 weeks of exercise (in rats) resulted in significantly increased levels of glutamic acid decarboxylase (GAD) mRNA transcripts (Kramer, Hahn, et al., 2002). GAD is the rate-limiting enzyme for GABA synthesis. These results suggest that exercise may have a direct effect on cardiovascular regulatory centers in the brain. Further research on mechanisms by which exercise exerts changes on neuronal function is needed.

Conclusion

The title of this chapter, "Impact of Exercise on Cognition in Older Adults: A Reexamination of Proposed Mechanisms," implies that we have more knowledge and a better understanding than we actually have of the complex physiological, neurophysiological, and chemical steps that translate the practice of strenuous exercise into a cognitively more efficient brain. This is particularly true for older people because the majority of pertinent research has focused on younger subjects.

Based on existing literature regarding animals and humans, it seems safe to assume that endurance exercise does improve cognitive function (see Dustman et al., 1994). As a result of neurophysiological adaptations to lifestyles of strenuous activity that have occurred over many millions of years, it should not be surprising that a linkage between exercise and cognition exists.

To efficiently and quickly respond to internal and external demands, the CNS must be able to react quickly and accurately. Because the brain does not store oxygen and glucose, which are essential for fueling the brain and enabling the metabolism of neurotransmitters, CBF and vasculature are necessary components of the response system. The brain is able to respond to neural demands for additional oxygen or glucose or both when these substrates are depleted by neuronal activity and is able to replenish them quickly and precisely to areas measured in μm (Silver, 1978). Autoregulation of the delivery of metabolic substrates is supported by vasoactive substances that constrict and dilate vessels and probably by nerve endings within the vessels themselves (Globus et al., 1983; Ide & Secher, 2000; Lou et al., 1987).

Efficient delivery of oxygen and glucose to the brain of older adults appears to be compromised by a slowing of CBF and by changes in blood characteristics that would restrict blood flow (Ajmani et al., 2000; Marchal et al., 1992; Slosman et al., 2001; Takada et al., 1992). These changes in CBF properties would be expected to impair cognitive functioning of older adults. However, physical activity appears to aid in the maintenance of cerebral perfusion into old age (Rogers et al., 1990).

Results of investigations of the immediate and somewhat longer effects of oxygen and glucose administration on cognitive functioning in laboratory settings provide illustrative examples of dynamic relationships between cognitive demand and brain perfusion. For example, investigators not only found that subjects' heart rates were elevated when cognitive tests were being performed (Scholey et al., 1999) but also that heart rate was positively related to task difficulty (Kennedy & Scholey, 2000). A more rapid heart rate would be expected to aid in the replenishing of oxygen and glucose depleted by high cognitive loads. Glucose ingestion was found to improve performance on tasks with a high cognitive demand but was less likely to affect performance on easy tests (Scholey et al., 2001; Winder & Borrill, 1998); blood glucose levels that were monitored during testing revealed greater reductions in glucose levels during difficult as compared to easier tasks (Scholey et al., 2001). Thus, it appears that baseline levels of oxygen and glucose are adequate for many of the routine activities performed each day and that, for more difficult cognitive tasks, physiochemical mechanisms within the cardiovascular system enable the delivery of additional metabolic substrates.

However, baseline levels of oxygen and glucose change as a function of age and aerobic fitness and would be expected to be considerably higher for young aerobically trained individuals than for old sedentary people. Thus, oxygen supplementation and glucose ingestion would be expected to have a more beneficial effect on cognitive performance of older than younger adults, in agreement with an earlier report (Hall et al., 1989). Similarly, sedentary subjects should receive a larger cognitive benefit from added oxygen or glucose or both than subjects who are aerobically fit and have higher baseline levels of these substances. Knowledge of fitness levels of subjects enrolled in studies of oxygen and glucose enrichment might well provide useful information for the interpretation of study results. For example, results following the administration of a standard dose of glucose to a sample of sedentary individuals might be different from results obtained from a sample of subjects of similar age who were physically more fit. On specific cognitive tasks, baseline levels of glucose might be adequate for good performance by physically active subjects who would thus not experience cognitive enhancement, while for less fit subjects, glucose supplementation could produce a significant improvement in cognitive performance. In studies of oxygen and glucose supplementation, information regarding fitness levels of experimental subjects should reduce unexplained variance between subjects and also decrease the number of conflicting reports regarding the effects of these metabolic substrates on cognition.

Measures of physical fitness would also seem appropriate for studies of cognition–inhibition relationships. Evidence cited earlier in this chapter strongly suggests that aerobic fitness is positively related to both inhibitory strength and cognition (for a review, see Dustman, Emmerson, & Shearer, 1996). Investigations of the interactions among aerobic status, cognition, and inhibition variables, particularly in studies of adult aging, should be interesting and should also identify sources of previously unknown between-subject variance and perhaps reconcile study results from different laboratories.

The research methodology described in the section, "Oxygen Administration and Cognition," provides a strong framework on which to base future studies of oxygen-cognition relationships. Oxygen inhalation during test administration had a positive effect on cognition of young adults (Moss & Scholey, 1996; Moss et al., 1998; Scholey et al., 1999; Scholey et al.,

1998); older adults were not studied. It seems reasonable to expect that the effects of oxygen inhalation on cognition would be larger for older adults who typically have lower blood oxygen saturation levels than young adults and would be larger for sedentary older individuals compared to those who are more physically fit. Such research should contribute to a better understanding of the relationship of mild anoxia to compromised cognitive function in older people.

Recent evidence that shows that physical exercise induces the expression of a brain-derived neurotrophic factor (BDNF) supports the hypothesis that decreases in cognitive function during aging may be closely related to decreases in activity levels among older adults. BDNF's relationship to estrogen depletion and hypertension also suggests that decreased physical activity may contribute significantly to cognitive changes after menopause and with aging. Further research on these and other issues will undoubtedly provide us with important and interesting information regarding interrelationships among physical activity, aging, and CNS efficiency.

The identification and understanding of mechanisms that intervene between physical activity and neurocognitive functioning are better understood today than they were a few years ago. It is certain that our understanding of these mechanisms and the interactions among them will be substantially improved during the next few years. However, it is important that this information be disseminated in an understandable fashion to public officials, health providers, and to the lay public to encourage greater participation in physical activity by people of all ages.

CHAPTER 5

Current Findings in Neurobiological Systems' Response to Exercise

Philip V. Holmes, PhD

As evidence of the beneficial effects of exercise on psychological well-being mounts, so too has interest in the neurobiological bases for these effects. In recent years, it has become increasingly clear that exercise promotes behavioral functioning by altering activity in discrete brain systems. Research has focused on the brain's monoaminergic neurotransmitters serotonin, norepinephrine, and dopamine because of the well-established role of these neurotransmitters in regulating cognitive processes, mood states, and disorders thereof. This chapter reviews the anatomy and functions of the brain systems implicated in the beneficial effects of exercise and discusses the impact of exercise on these systems. Although exercise undoubtedly influences activity throughout the central nervous system, the present review focuses on serotonergic projections of the raphe nuclei, the noradrenergic projections of the locus coeruleus, and the mesotelencephalic dopamine system. The effects of exercise on these monoamine neurotransmitter functions have been reviewed extensively in recent years (Dishman, 1997; Meeusen et al., 2001), and this chapter highlights some of the conclusions drawn in these previous reviews. The role of other neurotransmitter systems in exercise has been studied less extensively, and there is a major gap in our knowledge about the effects of exercise on the peptide neurotransmitters that coexist in monoaminergic neurons. The implications of recent findings concerning exercise-induced changes in peptidergic systems are explored.

This chapter also discusses the significance of recent evidence concerning the capacity for exercise to increase the synthesis of neurotrophic factors in the brain. Neurotrophic factors, such as brain-derived neurotrophic factor (BDNF), have been shown to enhance a variety of neuronal functions and protect neurons from degenerative processes or injury. Several investigators have proposed recently that BDNF may be the primary mediator of the beneficial effects of exercise on a range of psychological functions. Particular interest in BDNF's reversal of age-related decline has emerged in the past five years. Though the potential link between exercise and neurotrophin-mediated protection against neurodegeneration and age-related disease processes is an exciting new area of research, the experimental data supporting this link are still rather limited. Lacking thus far has been information concerning the neural mechanisms through which neurotrophic factors influence behavior. Nonetheless, the hypothetical link between exercise and long-term adaptations in neuronal structure and survival promises to be an important area for future investigation.

The final section of this chapter attempts to synthesize current findings on the neurobiological effects of exercise and proposes some specific neural mechanisms for exercise-induced improvements in psychological functioning. The models proposed are highly preliminary, and certain aspects of the mechanisms are speculative. The models are therefore intended more as heuristic tools to guide future research rather than formal explanations of extant data.

Neuroanatomical Systems Implicated in the Effects of Exercise

The following literature reviews demonstrate that exercise consistently alters activity in discrete neural systems in the brain. The majority of previous studies have focused on brain monoaminergic systems. Prior to the discussion of the neurobiological mechanisms underlying the effects of exercise on behavior, the neuroanatomy, biochemistry, and function of brain monoamine system will be briefly reviewed.

Mesotelencephalic Dopamine System

Projections of mesotelencephalic dopamine neurons originate from cell bodies located in the midbrain substantia nigra and ventral tegmental area. Though the projections from these adjacent nuclei overlap extensively, differential patterns of forebrain innervation exist. For example, substantia nigra neurons project more extensively to the dorsal striatum and piriform cortex, whereas ventral tegmental area neurons project predominantly to ventral striatal structures, the limbic system, and prefrontal cortex (Roth & Elsworth, 1995; Heimer, Zahm, & Alheid, 1995). The rate-limiting enzyme for dopamine synthesis is tyrosine hydroxylase (TH), which converts tyrosine to the dopamine precursor L-3,4-dihydroxyphenylalanine (DOPA). Dopamine receptor subtypes have been defined based on pharmacology and intracellular signaling pathways. The two major classes are commonly referred to as the D1-like and D2-like groups. The D1 group includes the subtypes D1 and D5, whereas the D2 group includes the subtypes D2, D3, and D4 (Seeman, 1995). The mesotelencephalic dopamine system is critically involved in motor control and initiation of movement, aversively and appetitively motivated behaviors, and reward. With respect to the latter function, several investigators have recently proposed that dopamine may be more involved in determining the incentive salience of stimuli (i.e., the desire for some stimulus) rather than the hedonics or pleasure associated with consummatory behavior (see Berridge & Robinson, 1998, for review).

Locus Coeruleus Norepinephrine System

The majority of forebrain axons that release norepinephrine originate from neurons in the locus coeruleus, a small cluster of cell bodies located in the pontine brainstem. The projections from the locus coeruleus are diffuse and far reaching, with particularly rich innervation of the olfactory bulb, frontal cortex, thalamus, hippocampus, and amygdala (Holmes & Crawley, 1995; Valentino & Aston-Jones, 1995). A noteworthy feature of locus coeruleus projections is the extent of collateralization: A single noradrenergic neuron may innervate several forebrain structures. This anatomical characteristic is consistent with the behavioral functions of this system, which involve regulation of arousal states, attention, and stress response (Foote & Aston-Jones, 1995). The locus coeruleus (LC)-norepinephrine system is thus poised to regulate cognitive activity by influencing a variety of brain systems in parallel. Noradrenergic receptors have been divided into the alpha and beta groups based primarily on their coupling with inhibitory or excitatory G-proteins, respectively. Several subtypes from each group have been identified based on differences in pharmacology and signal transduction pathways (Duman & Nestler, 1995). Like dopamine, the rate-limiting enzyme for norepinephrine synthesis is TH. Dopamine thus serves as a precursor for norepinephrine synthesis in noradrenergic neurons.

Raphe Nuclei Serotonin System

The anatomy of the ascending serotonergic innervation of the forebrain resembles that of the noradrenergic system. Projections are collateralized and even more extensive and far reaching than those of the noradrenergic system (Azmitia & Whitaker-Azmitia, 1995; Jacobs & Fornal, 1995). The majority of these projections originate in dorsal and median raphe nuclei and terminate in the substantia nigra, hippocampus, amygdala, olfactory bulb, and a variety of neocortical regions (Azmitia & Whitaker-Azmitia, 1995). The telencephalic serotonin system has been implicated in a range of behavioral functions, including motivational and emotional expression, hedonia, and impulse control (Jacobs & Fornal, 1995). At least 12 different serotonin receptor subtypes have been proposed (Sanders-Bush & Canton, 1995); and the behavioral complexity of the serotonin system reflects this pharmacological complexity. The rate-limiting enzyme of serotonin synthesis is tryptophan hydroxylase.

Neurochemical Adaptations to Exercise

Previous experiments have revealed widespread changes in neurotransmitters throughout the central nervous system. In reviewing these findings, it is important to consider methodological differences between studies. Postmortem analysis of tissue levels of a neurotransmitter is informative, but it provides less insight into function than do microdialysis techniques. Experiments examining exercise-induced changes in gene expression may provide the best indicator of long-term neuronal adaptations to exercise.

Monoamines

The influence of exercise on brain monoaminergic transmitters has been reviewed extensively by Dishman (1997) and Meeusen and colleagues (2001). Dishman's synthesis of the literature concerning exercise-induced changes in norepinephrine, serotonin, and their metabolites in the rat brain postmortem provides the following conclusions concerning exercise effects: Acute, low-intensity exercise (e.g., free access to an activity wheel) produces little or no change in brain monoamines measured postmortem using various fluometric or chromatographic techniques. Acute bouts of more intense exercise (e.g., forced treadmill running or forced swimming) generally increases monoamines and metabolites in several brain regions. Increased levels of norepinephrine and serotonin and their metabolites are more consistently observed in forebrain regions or whole-brain homogenates following chronic exercise. Decreases have also been observed in some brain regions. Although changes in these neurochemical markers have been reported by several groups, the nature of these changes (i.e., increase or decrease) and their neuroanatomical loci are highly variable and dependent on the nature and duration of exercise. As Dishman (1997) and Meeusen and colleagues (2001) point out, the differential effects of various modes of exercise must be considered when comparing studies. For example, though forced treadmill exercise may involve greater exertion than free running on an activity wheel, the former mode of exercise involves significant levels of stress. Thus, in the case of treadmill training, stress and exercise are seriously confounded. This particular problem represents one of the greatest challenges in exercise research using animal models. Cognizance of the differences in duration of exercise and the time course of the experimental paradigm overall is also critical for interpreting differences in findings across studies. Nonetheless, the data from postmortem analyses clearly indicate the involvement of monoaminergic systems in long-term neural adaptations to exercise.

Recent studies using microdialysis techniques in rats provide a more complete picture of the nature of the neurochemical sequelae of exercise, though some discrepancies with postmortem analyses are evident. The advantage of the microdialysis technique is that it permits repeated measurements through chronically implanted brain cannulae of neurotransmitters and their metabolites during the course of exercise. A recent review of microdialysis experiments in exercise rats by Meeusen and colleagues (2001) reveals the following general findings: Moderate- to high-intensity exercise (e.g., on a treadmill) acutely increases the release of dopamine, norepinephrine, serotonin, and their metabolites in the striatum. Serotonin release is also increased consistently in the hippocampus during exercise. Because most of the experiments reviewed by Meeusen and colleagues (2001) typically involved one to two weeks of training prior to the neurotransmitter measurements during exercise, it is difficult to determine whether the reported effects of exercise involve long-term adaptations to chronic activity or acute responses to exercise. A series of experiments conducted by Meeusen and colleagues (1997) help to resolve this issue. Rats were either trained on a treadmill or habituated to the apparatus for six weeks. Following this period, *in vivo* microdialysis measures of norepinephrine, dopamine, and glutamate in the rat striatum were conducted before and during an acute bout of treadmill exercise. Exercise acutely increased the release of these neurotransmitters equally in both groups, whereas the treadmill-trained rats exhibited lower basal levels of neurotransmitter release (Meeusen et al., 1997). These findings suggest that the long-term consequences of exercise involve decreases in monoaminergic neurotransmitter tone in the striatum.

Long-term activity-wheel exercise exerts a different pattern of effects on noradrenergic neurons in the frontal cortex. Soares and colleagues (1999) have reported that exercised and sedentary rats exhibit equivalent basal levels of norepinephrine release in the frontal cortex as measured by microdialysis. However, stress-induced norepinephrine release is blunted in exercised rats. These results indicate that although activity-wheel exercise may not alter basal levels of norepinephrine, some form of regulation occurs, which serves to inhibit the noradrenergic response to stress.

Studies of changes in the enzyme systems responsible for synthesizing monoamine transmitters reveal long-term adaptations to exercise that occur intracellularly. Approximately two weeks of treadmill training increases TH gene expression in the locus coeruleus and ventral tegmental area in rats (Tumer et al., 2001), although no changes in TH mRNA were observed following three weeks of activity-wheel running (Soares et al., 1999). As described earlier, the discrepancies between the two studies may be due to differences in exercise intensity, especially considering that the overall daily running distance tended to be comparatively low in the latter study. That exercise increases norepinephrine and dopamine biosynthetic capacities at the level of gene expression suggests that exercise produces relatively long-lasting and stable changes in these neurotransmitter systems. Chronic exercise also increases the activity and levels of tryptophan hydroxylase, the rate-limiting enzyme for serotonin synthesis, in the raphe nuclei (Chaouloff et al., 1987; Lim et al., 2001).

The analysis of receptor densities provides further evidence that exercise produces prolonged adaptations in monoamine neurotransmitters. Twelve weeks of treadmill training increases dopamine D2 receptor densities in the striatum (Gilliam et al., 1984). Similar increases in striatal dopamine receptor binding were observed following eight weeks of operantly conditioned wheel running for food reinforcement (DeCastro & Duncan, 1985). This receptor upregulation is consistent with exercise-induced decreases in the basal dopamine release described earlier. Treadmill training similarly protects against the decline in striatal dopamine receptors that occurs during aging (MacRae et al., 1987). This result was interpreted by the investigators as a neurotrophic effect of exercise. The relevance of this finding to recent evidence of exercise-induced elevations in brain neurotrophic molecules is discussed later.

Long-term treadmill training produces the desensitization of serotonergic 5-HT1B receptors in the substantia nigra (Chennaoui et al., 2000) and the decrease in levels of mRNA encoding in these receptors in the cerebellum and frontal cortex (Chennaoui et al., 2001). The sedative effects of the serotonin agonist 1-(3-chlorophenyl)piperazine (mCPP) are also diminished in treadmill-trained rats (Dwyer & Browning, 2000). These effects may reflect adaptations in serotonergic systems to repeated exercise-induced increases in serotonergic transmission.

Measures of metabolic activity similarly suggest long-term, intracellular adaptations to exercise. Six months of activity-wheel access increases levels of cytochrome oxidase, an enzyme involved in ATP production, in the frontal cortex and striatum (McCloskey, Adamo, & Anderson, 2001). These metabolic changes are probably initiated early during first exposure to the exercise paradigm; studies of acute locomotor activity reveal immediate changes in metabolic markers. For example, exercise acutely increases local cerebral glucose utilization, a putative marker of neuronal activity, in the striatum, motor cortex, and hippocampus (Vissing, Andersen, & Diemer, 1996). Acute treadmill exercise also increases expression of the immediate, early gene c-fos in the striatum, which is a marker of cellular transcriptional activity, and this effect is mediated by dopamine transmission via D-1 receptors (Liste et al., 1997).

Taken together, this evidence suggests that exercise acutely and tonically regulates the functions of norepinephrine, dopamine, and serotonin systems. Acute responses involve enhanced release of dopamine, norepinephrine, and serotonin in the forebrain. Long-term adaptations include decreased basal release of monoamines and increased receptor density, synthetic enzyme expression, and metabolic activity. Although these effects depend on the duration and intensity of the exercise, these monoaminergic alterations provide a likely explanation for some of the beneficial effects of exercise on psychological functions. Specific hypothetical mechanisms are discussed as follows.

Peptides

Although the influence of exercise on peptide hormone release by endocrine systems has been extensively studied (see Jonsdottir, 2000, for review), relatively little research has examined exercise-induced regulation of peptide neurotransmitters in the brain. A variety of peptides coexist with the monoamine transmitters in the systems described earlier. The mesolimbic dopamine system involves several peptide transmitters that mediate critical functions with respect to reward, locomotor activation, and stress responses. Examples include the opioid peptides enkephalin and dynorphin as well as cholecystekinin, and substance P (Deutch & Bean, 1995; Hokfelt et al., 2000). Cholecystekinin coexists with dopamine neurons of the substantia nigra and ventral tegmental area. The opioid peptides and substance P are primarily found in gamma amino butyric acid (GABA) neurons of the striatum that project to ventral pallidum or back to midbrain dopamine neurons (Heimer et al., 1995). In the noradrenergic system, galanin is the primary peptide coexisting with norepinephrine. Galanin is a 29 amino–acid peptide that is found in more than 80 percent of noradrenergic locus coeruleus neurons (Holmes & Crawley, 1995). Neuropeptide Y, a 36 amino–acid peptide, also coexists extensively in locus coeruleus neurons, although to a lesser extent than galanin (Holmes & Crawley, 1995). Galanin, neuropeptide Y, and other peptides are also expressed in serotonergic neurons in the raphe nuclei (Hokfelt et al., 2000).

O'Neal and coworkers have recently reported that exercise increases prepro-galanin mRNA levels in the LC (O'Neal et al., 2001). Another recent experiment, using microarray analysis of gene expression in the hippocampus, confirmed that exercise upregulates galanin gene expression in this structure as well (Tong et al., 2001). Other brain regions were not studied. Typical of gene array studies, the expression of many genes was found to be altered by exercise. However, a surprising outcome of this experiment was the observation that galanin was the only non-neurotrophin neurotransmitter system to be influenced by exercise (Tong et al., 2001). This finding suggests that galanin may play a prominent role in exercise effects. Because galanin influences appetitively and aversively motivated behaviors that are profoundly altered in clinical depression (e.g., sexual behavior, feeding, stress responses) and regulates several hypophysiotropic hormones in the hypothalamus, this peptide may be a critical mediator of the antidepressant and antistress effects of exercise (Bloch et al., 1998;

Corwin, Robinson, & Crawley, 1993; Gundlach & Burazin, 1998; Holmes & Crawley, 1995).

Access to activity wheels for 30 days increases dynorphin gene expression in the striatum of Lewis rats, a strain that exhibits high levels of voluntary running (Werme et al., 2000). This finding was interpreted in the context of endogenous opioid mediation of some of the rewarding or addictive properties of exercise. The role of endogenous opioid peptides in exercise has also been demonstrated through pharmacological manipulations. The opioid receptor antagonist naloxone causes a dose-dependent decrease in activity-wheel running, suggesting that activation of endogenous opioid systems is necessary for the initiation and maintenance of exercise (Sisti & Lewis, 2001). Activity-wheel running leads to sufficient activation of endogenous opioid systems to produce tolerance to the rewarding (Lett et al., 2002) and analgesic (Kanarek et al., 1998; Mathes & Kanarek, 2001) effects of morphine in rats, further supporting the hypothesis that endogenous opioid systems may mediate some exercise-induced behavioral adaptations.

Trophic Factors

The discovery that exercise increases the expression of neurotrophic factors in the brain has received considerable attention recently. Neurotrophic factors are neuronal proteins that function to maintain, protect, and promote growth in a variety of neuronal populations (Mufson et al., 1999). Prominent examples include brain-derived neurotrophic factor (BDNF), neurotrophin-3, and nerve growth factor (NGF), all three of which belong to a single neurotrophic factor gene family (Lewin & Bard, 1996). These neurotrophins have been shown to promote neuronal sprouting, axonal regeneration, and synapse formation (Lewin & Bard, 1996; McAllister, Katz, & Lo, 1999). Neurotrophins are released synaptically, and their cellular effects are mediated by tyrosine kinase receptors, which signal through a variety of intracellular mechanisms, including cyclic-AMP response element-binding protein (CREB) and mitogen-activated protein kinases (MAPK). Neurotrophins also influence neuronal function through retrograde or anterograde axonal transport. This process may be particularly important for neurotrophin mediation of neuronal development, differentiation, and repair (Mufson et al., 1999). The neurotrophins are expressed throughout the brain, though some of the highest levels are found in the hippocampus (Lewin & Bard, 1996; McAllister et al., 1999).

Several different laboratories, including ours, have demonstrated that providing free access to running wheels for seven days or more increases brain levels of BDNF in rats (Neeper et al., 1996; Russo-Neustadt et al., 2001; Van Hoomissen et al., 2004) These exercise-induced changes occur primarily in the hippocampus. Studies of gene expression using microarray techniques in the rat hippocampus have confirmed exercise-induced increases in various neurotrophins, including BDNF (Tong et al., 2001). Activity-wheel exercise similarly increases expression of CREB and MAPK, the intracellular signaling molecules for BDNF, in the hippocampus. Prolonged access to activity wheels also increase the expression of growth-associated protein-43, a marker of neurite outgrowth, and synaptophysin, a marker of synaptogenesis, in the hippocampus in mice (Chen et al., 1998). These results provide specific evidence for neurotrophin-mediated increases in neuronal sprouting and synapse formation. BDNF is particularly effective in promoting the sprouting of serotonergic neurons (Mamounas et al., 2000), which has been suggested as a basis for its potential antidepressant effects (Altar, 1999) (see the following discussion).

In addition to increasing the expression of neurotrophins in the brain, exercise increases levels of other types of trophic factors derived from endocrine tissues. Two weeks of treadmill running increases plasma levels of insulin-like growth factor-I in rats (Carro et al., 2001). The exercise-induced increase in circulating insulin-like growth factor-I protected against experimentally induced neurotoxicity, suggesting that this hormonal neurotrophic factor mediates some of the neuroprotective effects of exercise (Carro et al., 2001).

Beneficial Effects of Exercise on Psychological Functions: Basic Studies in Animal Models

The following section reviews several lines of evidence indicating that exercise exerts beneficial effects on a variety of psychological functions. These basic experiments provide a compelling rationale for further exploration of these beneficial effects in humans.

Antidepressant and Antistress Effects

The application of animal models is essential for studying the neurobiological basis for the antidepressant effects of exercise. The first and overriding criterion one must apply in selecting the appropriate animal model of depression to study how exercise exerts its antidepressant effects is whether exercise does indeed produce antidepressant-like effects in the model. The two models, neonatal clomipramine and olfactory bulbectomy, stand out in this regard. Because they involve long-lasting depression-related behavioral abnormalities that are reversed by exercise, the neonatal clomipramine and olfactory bulbectomy models show particular promise for studying the neurobiological mechanisms for the antidepressant effects of exercise. At the time of this writing, there is no published evidence that any other model of depression responds to exercise in this way. Although previous studies have demonstrated that exercise may mitigate the impact of stressors (see the following discussion), the models employed in these studies are better suited for examining the protective effects of exercise against the development of stress-induced depression rather than the therapeutic effects of exercise on reversing depression symptoms (Dishman, 1997; Moraska & Fleshner, 2001).

Previous work from the laboratory of Dishman has demonstrated that exercise exerts antidepressant-like effects in a rat model of depression induced by neonatal treatment with the serotonin reuptake inhibitor clomipramine (Yoo et al., 2000). This model produces long-lasting deficits in appetitively motivated behavior analogous to depression symptoms of anhedonia such as decreased sexual behavior, decreased consumption of highly palatable foods, and decreased intracranial self-stimulation (Vogel et al., 1990). Yoo and coworkers (2000) demonstrated that prolonged access to activity wheels reverses the deficits in sexual behavior that occur in the neonatal clomipramine model. More recent experiments from our laboratory demonstrate nearly identical effects of exercise in the olfactory bulbectomized rat model of depression (Chambliss et al., 2004). This model similarly involves deficits in appetitively motivated behavior and other "anhedonia-like" phenomena. Three weeks of activity-wheel exercise reversed the deficits in sexual behavior caused by olfactory bulbectomy (OBX).

The consistency of these results demonstrates convergence between the two models. Finding similar effects of exercise in two distinct animal models suggests that the capacity for exercise to reverse depression symptoms may be a general phenomenon. The results also demonstrate the independence of olfaction in the beneficial effects of exercise in the OBX model. Though deficits in sexual behavior in bulbectomized rats may involve anosmia to a certain extent, the restoration produced by exercise clearly is unrelated to olfaction because it is reasonable to assume that exercise did not restore olfactory functions. Previous research demonstrates that olfactory cues play an important role in sexual behavior, especially in its development, but olfaction is not necessary for the expression of sexual behavior (Larsson & Ahlenius, 1999).

Exercise may mitigate the impact of stress, thereby preventing the development of stress-related behavioral and physiological changes. Dishman and coworkers have provided extensive evidence demonstrating how exercise modifies endocrine stress responses. These changes include the enhancement of stress-induced adrenocorticotropic hormone (ACTH) and prolactin caused by chronic treadmill exercise (White-Welkley et al., 1996). Chronic activity-wheel exercise also blunts stress-induced norepinephrine release in the frontal cortex (Soares et al., 1999). These changes may reflect beneficial adaptations of the hypothalamic–pituitary and locus coeruleus norepinephrine systems, respectively, although the behavioral implications of these exercise-induced adaptations have yet to be elucidated. Moraska and Fleshner (2001) have demonstrated that exercise prevents the escape deficits that emerge in the learned helplessness model of stress and in stress-induced depression. Exercise thus prevents the development of behavioral abnormalities caused by severe, uncontrollable stress.

Although to date there is no evidence that exercise alone exerts antistress effects in other models of stress-induced depression, previous experiments have demonstrated that the combination of exercise and antidepressant administration reverses the immobility observed in the forced swim paradigm, which serves as a behavioral screening test for antidepressant drugs (Russo-Neustadt et al., 2001). This finding suggests that antidepressant pharmacotherapy and exercise may interact, possibly at the level of enhancing noradrenergic or serotonergic transmission, to alter acute stress responses. The possible role of BDNF in this effect is discussed later.

Neuroprotection

Previous research has demonstrated that exercise protects neurons against neuronal degeneration and death caused by ischemia (Stummer et al.,1995), neurotoxins (Carro et al., 2001), or excess free-radical activity (Radak et al., 2001). Although exercise has been shown to improve general behavioral functions in aging rats (Dorner et al., 1997; Skalicky, Bubna-Littitz, & Vidiik, 1996), the ability of exercise to slow or reverse age-related neural degeneration has yet to be conclusively established.

Learning

Extensive evidence of the ability of exercise to enhance cognitive functions in rats and mice has been reported, and such enhancement has been linked to specific changes in hippocampal functions (Anderson, Rapp, et al., 2000; Fordyce, Starnes, & Farrar, 1991; van Praag et al., 1999). For example, exercise improves performance in the radial-arm maze in rats (Anderson, Rapp, et al., 2000) and Morris water maze in mice (van Pragg et al., 1999). The exercise-induced improvements in mice were associated with increased hippocampal long-term potentiation, a putative physiological marker of learning. Activity-wheel running in mice also enhanced neurogenesis in the hippocampus, suggesting that exercise leads to the formation of new neurons in some brain regions (van Pragg et al., 1999).

Recent studies from our laboratory have demonstrated that activity-wheel exercise improved aversively motivated contextual learning in rats. The exercise-induced enhancement in learning was reversed by chronic administration of a beta-adrenergic receptor antagonist (Van Hoomissen et al., 2004). This result suggests that projections of locus coeruleus norepinephrine system are critical for the cognition-enhancing effects of exercise.

Hypothetical Models Linking Neurobiological and Behavioral Effects of Exercise

Figure 5.1 summarizes some of the current evidence regarding the relationship between exercise, neurobiological changes, and behavior. Although the data provide compelling explanations for the long-term behavioral effects of exercise, particularly with respect to neurotrophic factors, serious gaps are still evident. The most serious gap occurs between the increased neurotrophin expression and psychological functions. The ability of neurotrophic factors to increase sprouting and synaptogenesis is well established. The link between these forms of plasticity and behavior is also fairly solid. The questions that remain for the sake of understanding exercise's influence on behavior concern (1) the causality between these hypothetical links, (2) the specific paths through which exercise influences behavior, and (3) the relative contributions of these processes.

Another serious limitation in our understanding of the neurobiological basis of exercise-induced behavioral change is the lack of neuroanatomical evidence. Which brain systems mediate the beneficial effects and how? The evidence reviewed implicates the hippocampus as well as the mesotelencephalic dopamine system, the locus coeruleus norepinephrine system, the raphe nuclei serotonin system, and peptides coexisting in these pathways, but these systems are implicated only to the extent that neurochemical changes have been observed in them. With the possible exception of BDNF-induced enhancement of hippocampal long-term potentiation, missing are most of the specific links between exercise, neurobiological changes, the neuroanatomical systems involved, and behavior.

Novel hypotheses concerning the role of neural atrophy and degeneration in depression and other stress-related disorders have emerged recently (Altar, 1999; Duman et al., 1997; Rajkowska, 2000). These hypotheses are based on evidence of prolonged stress causing neuronal loss, decreased cellular densities, and decreased brain volumes in depressed individuals. The hypotheses propose that the neuronal degeneration caused by stress and depression may be reversed by interventions that increase endogenous neurotrophin activity. Several investigators have proposed that the antidepressant effects of exercise may be mediated in part by increased BDNF expression (Altar, 1999; Cotman and Berchtold, 2002; Cotman and Engesser-Cesar, 2002; Duman et al., 1999; Rajkowska, 2000). More specifically, BDNF may reverse the loss of hippocampal neurons that is putatively caused by stress and depression. This hypothesis has yet to be specifically tested in animal models of depression. A recent study by (Shirayama et al., 2002) provides some preliminary support for the hypothesis that BDNF may mitigate the deleterious impact of stress. Intrahippocampal injections of BDNF produce antidepressant effects in the forced swim and learned

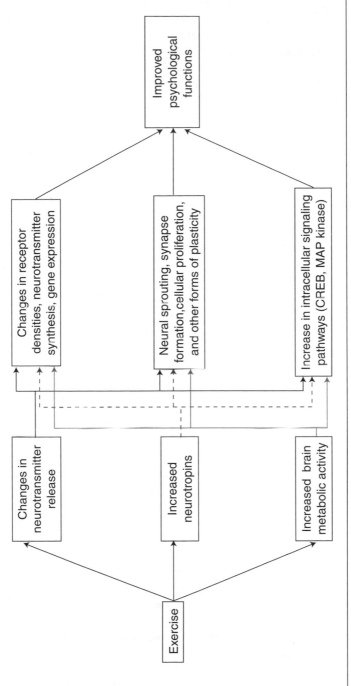

Figure 5.1 Exercise-induced protection against stress- and depression-related hippocampal degeneration.

helplessness models of stress (Shirayama et al., 2002). The relevance of these findings to the neurodegenerative hypothesis is unclear because hippocampal degeneration is not likely to occur in these paradigms given the brief interval between stress and subsequent behavioral testing (1-3 d). However, BDNF may produce its antistress effects in this model by enhancing activity in serotonergic neurons. Antidepressant-like effects of BDNF have also been observed following injections into the midbrain, suggesting that the effects of BDNF are not limited to the hippocampus but may be mediated by several different sites and possibly different neurotransmitters (Siuciak et al., 1997).

The hypotheses presented earlier propose that exercise-induced increases in BDNF produce acute antistress effects by modulating serotonergic transmission and protect against stress-induced hippocampal degeneration through its trophic actions. The first hypothesis has been supported empirically (Russo-Neustadt et al., 2001; Shirayama et al., 2002), but the other hypothesis has yet to be tested. Another major question that needs to be answered concerns the mechanism for chronic exercise elevating BDNF in the hippocampus. Exercise-induced increases in serotonergic and noradrenergic activity are good candidates. The hippocampus is densely innervated by serotonergic and noradrenergic neurons, and several lines of evidence reveal that neurotrophin levels are regulated by monoamine neurotransmitters (Russo-Neustadt et al., 1999).

Exercise-Induced Reversal of Deficits in Appetitively Motivated Behavior

Studies are currently underway in our laboratory to examine the neural mechanisms responsible for the antidepressant-like actions of exercise. In collaboration with Dishman and coworkers, we have focused on the deficits in male sexual behavior that occur in rat models of depression as an index of anhedonia-like phenomena. Recent experiments from our laboratory reveal that both treadmill and activity-wheel exercise cause long-term elevations in galanin gene expression in the locus coeruleus (O'Neal et al., 2001; Van Hoomissen et al., 2004). The increased expression of galanin in the LC may reverse some depression-related behavioral deficits. The behavioral functions of galanin include promotion of sexual behavior and feeding (Bloch et al., 1998; Corwin et al., 1993; Gundlach & Burazin, 1998; Holmes & Crawley, 1995). Galanin-containing LC neurons may directly stimulate sexual behavior by acutely activating hypothalamic circuits. This mechanism could involve the extensive projections of galaninergic neurons to the paraventricular nucleus (PVN) (Gundlach & Burazin, 1998; Holets et al., 1988). Although not extensively studied, galanin has been shown to stimulate prolactin secretion (Bloch et al., 1998; Gopalan et al., 1993), which may be mediated by galanin influences on hypophysiotropic factors in PVN neurons. Prolactin enhances reproductive behaviors in male rats (Cruz-Casallas et al., 1999; Drago & Lissandrello, 2000; Seal et al., 2000). This mechanism provides another explanation for how increased galanin synthesis in the LC may promote sexual behavior. Galaninergic neurons of the LC also project to the dopamine neurons of the ventral tegmental area. Although galanin administration into the ventral tegemental area acutely inhibits dopaminergic neurons (Weiss et al., 1998), long-term changes in galanin transmission caused by chronic exercise may exert opposite effects through receptor regulation. Galanin may thus enhance dopaminergic tone in the mesolimbic system over the long run, thereby increasing the expression of appetitively motivated behaviors.

Conclusion

Several lines of evidence reveal that neurotrophins play a critical role in learning and memory in several species (Johnston & Rose, 2001; Ma et al., 1998; Szabo & Hoffman, 1995). The effect of BDNF in enhancing hippocampal long-term potentiation provides a well-substantiated mechanism for understanding the neurobiological basis of exercise effects on cognition (Ma et al., 1998). The capacity for exercise to increase neurogenesis in the hippocampus (van Praag et al., 1999) provides another potential mechanism in which neurotrophins may enhance cognition. As described earlier, further studies are needed in order to determine which systems are responsible for mediating exercise-induced increases in hippocampal neurotrophins. Monoamine systems are an obvious starting point. The recent findings from our laboratory that the enhancement in contextual learning caused by exercise is blocked by a noradrenergic antagonist implicates norepinephrine. However, the role of neurotrophins in this process, if any, has yet to be established.

CHAPTER 6

Measurement of Physical Activity

Rod K. Dishman, PhD

Physical activity is defined as "any bodily movement produced by skeletal muscle that results in energy expenditure" (Caspersen, Powell, & Christenson, 1985, p. 126). It can occur as short, strenuous bursts or as less intense effort sustained over a longer period (Montoye, Kemper, Saris, & Washburn, 1996), and it includes occupational activity, chores, leisure activity, sports, and exercise that is planned for fitness or health purposes. Physical activity is the most variable component of an individual's total daily energy expenditure, which, in addition to voluntary physical activity, consists of basal metabolic rate and the thermic effect of food digestion. The large variability in daily physical activity within and among people in free-living populations makes the assessment of physical activity very difficult (Montoye & Taylor, 1984).

The valid assessment of physical activity has often been ignored in studies of physical activity and aging. Although the frequency, duration, and intensity of acute physical activity in a laboratory or clinical setting can be measured objectively by observation and physiological recordings, the causes and impact of physical activity on public health cannot be understood unless physical activity in free-living, unsupervised settings is measured. Current population estimates based on self-reports suggest that physical activity declines linearly with increasing age; older adults are markedly less active in most forms of physical activity than young and middle-aged adults. As depicted in figures 6.1, 6.2, and 6.3, among U.S. adults age 65 to 74 years, 51 percent report no leisure-time physical activity. Only 13 percent report vigorous physical activity sufficient to affect cardiorespiratory fitness, and 10 percent report engaging in resistance-type exercise for muscular strength or endurance. Comparable rates among people age 75 years or older are 65 percent for inactivity, 6 percent for vigorous physical activity, and 7 percent for resistance-type exercise (Centers for Disease Control & Prevention, 2001; U.S. Department of Health & Human Services, 2000).

The decline in physical activity with age seems to be less for moderately intense activities, as shown in figure 6.4. However, population estimates of physical activity in the United States have been based on questions not yet directly validated by comparisons with objective measures of physical activity. Hence, their accuracy has not been confirmed (Caspersen, Merritt, & Stephens, 1994) especially among older people, some of whom may represent unique measurement problems because of age-related changes in the types

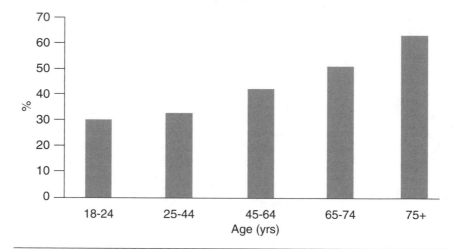

Figure 6.1 The percentage of adults who engage in no leisure-time physical activity.

From U.S. Department of Health & Human Services 2000.

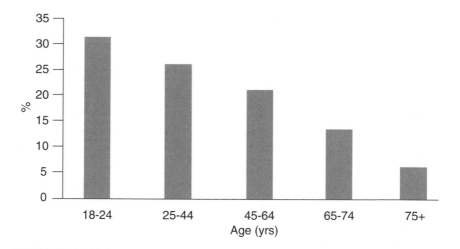

Figure 6.2 The percentage of adults who engage in vigorous physical activity that promotes cardiorespiratory fitness for 20 or more minutes, three or more days a week.

From U.S. Department of Health & Human Services 2000.

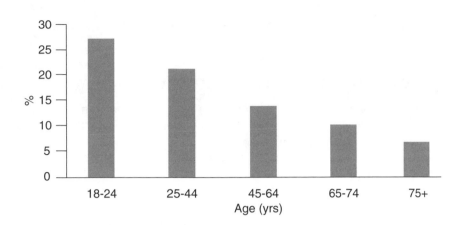

Figure 6.3 The percentage of adults who perform physical activities that enhance and maintain muscular strength and endurance.

From U.S. Department of Health & Human Services 2000.

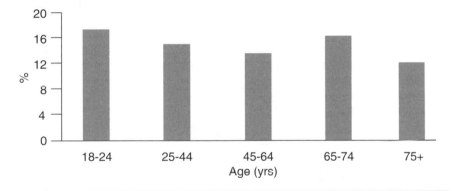

Figure 6.4 The percentage of adults who engage regularly, preferably daily, in moderate physical activity for at least 30 minutes per day.

From U.S. Department of Health & Human Services 2000.

and timing of their physical activities or declines in memory or gait that can affect the validity of self-reports or some motion-monitoring devices.

To determine the causes and functional or health outcomes of physical activity among older people, valid methods of assessing physical activity are required that are reliable (i.e., objective, accurate, and precise), nonobtrusive, and practical to administer. The purpose of this chapter is to discuss the approaches that have been taken to objectively estimate physical activity and its specific components and to determine whether self-reports are valid measures of physical activity. Although the measurement of physical activity among free-living people has a long history, traceable to a pedometer designed by Leonardo da Vinci nearly 500 years ago, it represents a persistent conundrum in the fields of epidemiology and clinical medicine. Today there is still no consensus "gold standard" for the measurement of physical activity.

Methods of Physical Activity Assessment

More than a dozen methods for measuring physical activity are currently available. The basic characteristics of these methods are presented in table 6.1 according to their appropriateness for use in a population, characterizing study costs, extent of interference with usual activity level, participant acceptability, and the ability of the method to provide specific information about the type, frequency, duration, and intensity of physical activity (LaPorte, Montoye, & Caspersen, 1985). These methods can also be categorized according to whether they provide a direct or indirect (e.g., self-report) observation of physical activity or assess body motion, a physiological response during physical activity, energy expenditure, or a physiological adaptation to physical activity.

Observation

Direct observation of physical activity can provide specific information about activity type, frequency, and duration but cannot measure physical activity intensity, either in terms of energy expenditure or relative physiological strain. A visual record can permit the rate of energy expenditure to be estimated by the computation of displacement of body mass and limb accelerations. Electronic surveillance is practical in some settings, although it may not be socially acceptable. Technologies such as global positioning satellite systems and body-mounted cameras are beginning to be used for physical activity assessment. Nonetheless, observation is usually impractical for a population study, is expensive, and can alter usual activity if people are aware that they are being observed.

Self-Reports

In the mid-1960s Henry J. Montoye quantified both the occupational and leisure-time physical activity habits recalled by participants using a questionnaire interview for use in the Tecumseh Michigan Community Health Study (Montoye, 1975). Since that time more than 30 physical activity survey questionnaires have been developed. Surveys of physical activity provide an indirect assessment of behavior based on self-reports by participants and rank highly on criteria of acceptability, cost, practicality, low interference with usual habits, and potential to provide specific activity information, except intensity. Physical activity questionnaires differ widely, however, on accuracy. An activity diary (i.e., a contemporaneous record of physical activity) can be very accurate about type, frequency, and duration when faithfully maintained. But, as

Table 6.1   Methods Used to Assess Physical Activity

| Assessment procedure | Study costs | | | Acceptability | | Activity specifics |
	Time	Effort	Interference	Personal	Social	
Calorimetry						
Direct	VH	VH	H-VH	No	No	Yes
Indirect	H-VH	VH	H-VH	No	No	Yes
Surveys						
Task-specific diary	L-M	L-M	VH	?	Yes	Yes
Recall questionnaire	L-M	L-M	L	Yes	Yes	Yes
Quantitative history	L-M	L-M	L	Yes	Yes	Yes
Physiologic markers						
Cardiorespiratory fitness	M-VH	M-H	L	?	?	No
Doubly labeled water	H-VH	M-VH	L-H	Yes	Yes	No
Mechanical and electronic monitors						
Heart rate	H-VH	M-VH	L-M	Yes	Yes	No
Pedometers	L-M	L	L-M	Yes	Yes	No
Accelerometers	L-H	L-M	L-M	Yes	Yes	No
Observation	H-VH	H-VH	L-VH	?	?	Yes

H = high; VH = very high; L = low; M = moderate

Adapted from LaPorte et al. 1985.

a surrogate for observation, a diary can motivate people to become more active during the time being studied.

A recall survey avoids the problems of interference with usual activity, but its accuracy varies according to the length of time being recalled and the complexity or regularity of people's habits. In addition, there is a tendency for people to overestimate their physical activity level. The longer the period of recall, the greater is the potential for capturing a person's true habits, but the greater also the risk that memory will be inaccurate. A sedentary person and a person who has a routine pattern of activity each should be able to accurately remember their habits, whereas a person who is sporadically active will likely not be as accurate in recollection. Despite their practical appeal, self-ratings of physical activity remain inherently flawed because they depend on a person's ability and motivation to report accurately. Notwithstanding the inherent imperfection of questionnaires, in many circumstances they represent the most valid option for measuring all features of physical activity in a feasible and cost-effective manner. Self-reports may be as accurate in ranking large groups of people according to level of physical activity as other more objective measures despite flaws in their ability to accurately measure the absolute level of physical activity.

Descriptions of more than 30 survey questionnaires for the measurement of physical activity and information about their reliability and validity have been published elsewhere (Pereira et al., 1997; Montoye et al., 1996; Washburn & Montoye, 1986). These questionnaires differ on several important factors such as the time frame over which activity is assessed (past week to lifetime), type of activity assessed (leisure, household, transportation, occupation), length, administration mode (interview or self administered), and outcome measure (Kcal, MET-hrs, unit-less score). Although several of these measures have been used with older people, they were not designed or validated for that purpose, and they may not be sensitive or specific enough to accurately assess some types or features of physical activities common among older people.

Examples of self-report measures of physical activity used in some influential clinical and population-based studies illustrate some of the potential problems of assessing physical activity among older people. The Physicians' Health Study was a randomized, double-blind, placebo-control trial designed to determine if low-dose aspirin decreases the risk for coronary heart disease and if beta-carotene decreases the risk for both coronary heart disease and cancer. Physical activity in this study was assessed by the question, "How often do you exercise vigorously enough to work up a sweat?" Response categories were "daily," "five to six times per week," "two to four times per week," "once a week," "one to three times per month," or "rarely/never." There is some evidence for the validity of this item as an indicator of physical activity level (Siconolfi et al., 1985; Washburn et al., 1990), and activity assessed with the sweat question has been associated with health outcomes (Manson et al., 1992). However, this item assesses a very specific type of physical activity, which may be engaged in by only a small and highly select segment of the older population. The Nurses' Health Study is a prospective study of health and lifestyle factors in 121,700 female registered nurses begun in 1976. In addition to other types of leisure-time physical activity, respondents were asked to report the average amount of time spent each week during the past year in walking or hiking outdoors and to estimate their usual walking pace as easy or casual, average, brisk, or very brisk. The validity and reliability of self-reports of walking distance and speed has not been established, especially among older people who likely differ more than do people of younger ages.

Only a few established physical activity surveys are designed for use among people older than 65 years; descriptions of four of them follow: (1) Modified Baecke Questionnaire for Older Adults, (2) Physical Activity Scale for the Elderly, (3) Yale Physical Activity Survey for Older Adults, and (4) Zutphen Physical Activity Questionnaire. Physical activity surveys specific to women and ethnic minorities or that assess specific features of physical activity that may be related to specific health outcomes or activities that increase muscular strength have not yet been developed. It is generally thought that individuals tend to overestimate participation in vigorous-intensity activities and underestimate participation in light to moderate activities (Sallis & Saelens, 2000), but this hasn't been confirmed among older people. Further research is also needed about ways to enhance people's recall of physical activities according to their intensity.

SELF-REPORT MEASURES OF PHYSICAL ACTIVITY DESIGNED FOR USE WITH OLDER ADULTS

Modified Baecke Questionnaire for Older Adults

Voorrips, L.E., A.C.J. Revelli, P.C.A. Dongelmans, P. Deurenberg, and W.A. Van Stavern. (1991). A physical activity questionnaire for the elderly. *Medicine and Science in Sports and Exercise, 23,* 974-979.

Content and Format (Past Yr, Recall Interview)

- 4-level ratings of household, sport, and leisure activities coded according to METs

Validity Evidence

- 31 free-living men and women age 63 to 80 years
- Correlations: repeated 24-hr recalls, $r = 0.78$; 3 d pedometer counts, $r = 0.72$

(continued)

(continued)

Physical Activity Scale for the Elderly (PASE)

Washburn, R.A., K.W. Smith, A.M. Jette, and C.A. Janney. (1993). The Physical Activity Scale for the Elderly (PASE): Development and evaluation. *Journal of Clinical Epidemiology, 46,* 153-162.

Content and Format (Past 7 d, Recall Interview or Self-Rating)

- 4-level ratings of leisure-time activities; summation of yes–no response for household and work-related activities coded according to regression weights from principal components analysis

Validity Evidence

- 222 free-living men and women age 65 and older
- Correlations: heart rate (HR), $r = -0.13$; grip strength, $r = 0.37$; static balance, $r = 0.33$; leg strength, $r = 0.25$

Yale Physical Activity Survey for Older Adults

DiPietro, L., C.J. Caspersen, A.M. Ostfeld, and E.R. Nadel. (1993). A survey for assessing physical activity among older adults. *Medicine and Science in Sports and Exercise, 25,* 628-642.

Content and Format (1 Mo, Recall Interview)

- MET $\cdot$ h $\cdot$ wk^{-1} for work, yard work, caretaking, exercise, and recreational activities; vigorous index; walking index; summary indexes: total time (h/wk); energy expenditure (Kcal/wk); activity dimensions

Validity Evidence

- 14 men and 11 women age 60 to 86 years
- Correlations: est $\dot{V}O_2$peak vs. total time index, $r = 0.58$; vs. vigorous index, $r = 0.60$; Caltrac counts vs. Kcal/wk, $r = 0.14$; vs. total time index, $r = 0.37$; vs. vigorous index, $r = 0.14$; vs. leisure walking index, $r = 0.31$

Zutphen Physical Activity Questionnaire

Caspersen, C.J., B.P.M. Bloemberg, W.H.M. Saris, R.K. Merritt, and D. Kromhout. (1991). The prevalence of selected physical activities and their relation with coronary heart disease risk factors in elderly men. *American Journal of Epidemiology, 133,* 1078-1092.

Westerterp, K.R., W.H.M. Saris, B.P.M. Bloemberg, K. Kempen, C.J. Caspersen, and D. Kromhout. (1992). Validation of the Zutphen Physical Activity Questionnaire for the elderly with doubly labeled water. *Medicine and Science in Sports and Exercise, 24,* S68.

Content and Format (Past wk, past mo, or usual, self-rated)

- MET $\cdot$ h $\cdot$ d^{-1} or Kcal $\cdot$ h $\cdot$ d^{-1} computed from list of 27 hobbies and sports.

Validity Evidence

- 21 free-living Dutch men age 70 to 89 years
- Correlations: Monthly total hours of physical activity vs. energy expenditure (EE) estimated from doubly labeled water/MET, $r = 0.61$

Biological Markers

In the same way that a self-report can be used to corroborate or provide specific information to complement objective estimates of physical activity, some degree of objective verification is required to corroborate the accuracy and validity of self-reports of physical activity. Methods for directly measuring energy expenditure in a lab are the most accurate but require a metabolic chamber, are limited to use with very small groups, apply to a limited number of types of activities, and are too costly for population studies. Also, they require simultaneous observation of activity in order to provide specific information about how the energy was expended (i.e., type, frequency, duration, and intensity). A measure of oxygen consumption is a slightly less accurate way to estimate energy expenditure using indirect calorimetry that is more practical because it permits usual activities to be performed outside a laboratory. However, this approach is also expensive (each monitor costs about $35,000), interferes with usual activities, and does not provide specifics about the physical activity. The use of doubly labeled water to estimate energy expenditure outside a laboratory offers a feasible and unobtrusive approach for large numbers of people, but it is expensive ($500-$800 per person), is susceptible to several types of error (though less than 10 percent error is possible in field studies), and does not indicate periodic changes in the rate of energy expenditure or type of physical activity.

Heart rate recorders provide surrogate measures of energy expenditure (with 5-25% errors depending on type of activity) and intensity, respectively, that are less costly (about $300-$600 per unit) and more practical. They also can indicate time, which permits a measure of the frequency, duration, and rate with which physical activities are carried out. However they do not give specifics about the type of physical activity; they require observation or self-report to corroborate the types and amounts of physical activity that occurred. Also, they may motivate people to increase their physical activity beyond usual because they are a type of observation. Also, recorders can malfunction, they might be removed without the knowledge of the investigator, and factors other than movement can elevate heart rate.

Physical fitness can be measured with only 2 to 3 percent error and offers an objective approach to indicating physical activities indirectly, assuming that a change in fitness has resulted from biological adaptations resulting from physical activity. Different types of fitness require specific types and rates of physical activity. Therefore, a measurement of fitness level provides an indirect way of inferring participation in activities that differ in cardiorespiratory, muscular, and flexibility demands. Similarly, changes in fitness depend on the amount or the rate of activities, so they also permit an approximation of specific dose-response relationships between physical activity participation and risk of specific diseases without observation of physical activity. Also, measures of fitness can be practically implemented in population studies. However, fitness is an attribute of a person, not a behavior. For example, about 30 percent of aerobic fitness is explainable by genetic expression (Perusse et al., 1989). That genetic influence on fitness, relative to the influence of physical activity, seems to diminish substantially as people age. For example, among young children cardiorespiratory fitness (i.e., $\dot{V}O_2$peak) changes more with the rate of maturation than with exercise training. By middle age, however, decreased cardiovascular fitness is mainly explainable by physical inactivity and weight gain. Hence, fitness is a good estimate of physical activity among adults who do not have a physical limitation to fitness testing. Nonetheless, certain aspects of physical activity may be very important in specific diseases or healthy functions (e.g., weight bearing activity such as walking for agility or stretching exercises for full range of joint motion) but not be reflected in a test of cardiorespiratory fitness, such as a maximal treadmill endurance test.

Direct Calorimetry

The most precise measure of energy expenditure available is direct calorimetry. In this method a person remains in an enclosed chamber while being studied, and caloric expenditure is determined by the production of heat (1 Kcal of energy is equivalent to an elevation in temperature of 1 kg of water by 1 degree Celsius). Direct calorimetry is highly accurate to less than 1 percent error. Direct calorimetry obviously limits normal activity; therefore, its value lies as a highly accurate tool to validate other physical activity assessment methods.

Indirect Calorimetry

Indirect calorimetry involves measuring the consumption of oxygen by analyzing expired air. This technique can be used in a metabolic chamber, which permits the measurement of the concentrations of oxygen and carbon dioxide in the room air. A less restrictive approach requires that the person wear a mask or a mouthpiece and nose clip while expired air is collected and then analyzed for gas concentrations. The participant must carry a gas collection container or remain within the confines of a laboratory or near remote sensors. The respiratory quotient is used to estimate caloric expenditure (e.g., the caloric equivalent is about 5 Kcal . L^{-1} . min^{-1} O_2 on a typical mixed diet). Error reported in indirect calorimetry is 2 to 3 percent.

Although more practical than direct calorimetry, this method still limits normal activity patterns. A portable gas analyzer weighing less than 1 kg was introduced about 10 years ago. This system (Cosmed K4b^2, Rome, Italy) contains a flow meter and a capillary tube for sampling expired air. Gas is analyzed by a small polarographic electrode. An FM transmitter carried by the person broadcasts signals to a receiver unit up to 600 meters away. When calibrated properly, this device provides estimates of $\dot{V}O_2$ within about 1.5 ml . kg^{-1} . min^{-1} of measures obtained by gas analysis using standard Douglas bag collection at seated rest and during cycling power outputs ranging from 50 to 200 W (Bassett, 2000). It allows researchers to validate other physical activity assessment methods without unduly restricting normal activity.

Dietary Measures

For this method to be valid, very precise records of caloric intake must be kept. The assumption is made that if an individual is maintaining a stable weight, caloric intake will be an accurate indication of energy expenditure. Even if a person's weight changes during the measurement period, caloric expenditure can still be estimated if precise body weight and body composition records are kept. Furthermore, the assumption is made that all persons are equally efficient in absorbing nutrients from the digestive tract. Typically, there is considerable error between recalled dietary intakes and actual food intakes measured by investigators. The use of dietary intake to estimate physical activity should occur over many days in controlled settings (Black, 1996). Weighing and recording food portions appears to be too demanding to expect adherence among most people in their natural environment.

Doubly Labeled Water (DLW)

The DLW method is currently the preferred method for determining energy requirements of healthy and clinical populations (Schoeller, 1999). In this method, a person drinks a prescribed dose of water containing isotopic hydrogen and oxygen. These tracers convert the body water into a virtual metabolic recorder that integrates H_2O output and CO_2 production for the next 7 to 14 days. By collecting urine during this period, these rates can be measured without the burden of collecting respiratory gases. Total energy expenditure can be estimated from CO_2 production.

The technique was first developed by Nathan Lifson and colleagues at the University of Minnesota in the late 1950s after they observed that the oxygen exhaled in CO_2 was in isotopic equilibrium with the oxygen in water during a series of experiments designed to determine whether the source of oxygen in expired CO_2 was molecular oxygen (Lifson et al., 1949). When a person drinks a measured dose of water labeled with the stable isotopes ^2H and ^{18}O, these two labels quickly distribute in body water and start to be eliminated from the body. The ^2H is eliminated from the body as ^2HHO, and the ^{18}O is eliminated as $H_2^{18}O$ and $C^{18}O_2$. The ^2H elimination is a measure of H_2O flux, while the ^{18}O elimination is a measure of H_2O and CO_2 flux. The difference between the two elimination rates is therefore a measure of CO_2 flux. The initial isotope enrichment and the fraction of each isotope remaining in the body at any time during the 7 to 14 days after the dose can be measured in the urine and the elimination rates calculated.

The initial validations of the method were also performed by Lifson and coworkers in rodent models as summarized by Lifson and McClintock (1966), and the feasibility for human use was proposed in 1975 (Lifson, Little, Levitt, & Henderson). The first human validation was reported in 1982 (Schoeller & van Santen). Since then, validations have been performed by multiple investigators. As reviewed by Schoeller (1988), validations against 4 to 5 days of respiratory gas exchange or 14 days of measured energy intake have demonstrated an accuracy of 1 to 2 percent and precision of 4 to 8 percent under most conditions.

The method, however, is sensitive to small errors in the isotopic analysis and interference from natural variations in these two stable isotopes. These errors reduce the precision. This sensitivity is a consequence of the nature of the method. Because the energy expenditure is calculated from the difference between ^2H and ^{18}O elimination rates and because that difference is between one-fourth to one-fifth of the tracer elimination rate, an error of 2 percent in the tracer elimination rate results in an 8 to 10 percent error in the estimated energy expenditure. Although the best laboratories have minimized analytical error and can yield estimates of energy expenditure having errors of only 3 to 6 percent, errors in excess of 30 percent have been reported (Roberts et al., 1995). Similarly, fluctuations in the background abundances of the naturally occurring ^2H and ^{18}O typically alter precision by a few percent; errors can be quite large if subjects are exposed to a new source of drinking water that has a different isotopic natural abundance as would occur if a person traveled during the measurement period (Horvitz & Schoeller, 2001). Other sources of error in the DLW method (Prentice, 1990) include: (1) a systematic change in body water of 4 percent, which can be estimated from acute changes in weight, results in an error in total energy expenditure of 2 percent; (2) loss of tracer atoms from body water other than as H_2O or CO_2 (e.g., incorporation of ^2H into fat synthesis in an amount equivalent to 20 percent of energy expenditure introduces an error of 5 percent); and (3) errors in the estimate of respiratory quotient (RQ) used in calculating energy expenditure introduce a 1 percent error for each 0.01 RQ unit.

The advantages of the doubly labeled water include: (1) objectivity, (2) use of stable isotopes, (3) its noninvasive nature, (4) length of the assessment period (7-14 d), and (5) the ease with which it can be used in free-living subjects. The disadvantages include: (1) high cost ($500 for a single dose of ^{18}O), (2) the need for expensive isotope ratio mass spectrometry and experienced technical support, (3) the fact that a measure of CO_2 production rather than O_2 consumption is obtained, and (4) the fact that it measures total energy expenditure and not physical activity or intensity or frequency of physical activity.

Although use of the doubly labeled water technique has become common in studies of energy expenditure during physical activity (Westerterp, de Boer, Saris, Schoffelen, & Ten Hoor, 1984; Westerterp, Brouns, Saris, & Ten Hoor, 1988; Westerterp, 1998), its primary value remains as a tool for validating less costly field methods for the assessment of physical activity that also provide specific features of physical activity (e.g., Gretebeck, Montoye, & Porter, 1991.) Examples include heart rate monitors and motion sensors.

Heart Rate Monitors

A variety of heart rate monitors using chest or other electrode placements are commercially available. The most valid and accurate monitors are those that measure electrical activity of the heart with conventional chest electrodes. The Polar heart rate monitor (Polar Electro Oy, Kempele, Finland) has become the most popular commercial monitor used in the United States. It is a cordless portable heart rate monitor that consists of a transmitter and a receiver. The transmitter weighs 43 grams or less and is attached to the chest either with an elastic belt that has built-in electrodes or with self-adhesive electrodes. The receiver (30-40 g) is also a digital wristwatch and contains a microcomputer for storing heart rate and time values. Both units are powered by lithium batteries. A heart rate monitor that records R-R intervals every 5, 15, or 60 seconds up to 133 hours and is PC compatible costs about $400. The PC-compatible software costs $200.

Correlations between the heart rate monitor and electrocardiographic recordings of heart rate are about 0.95 to 0.97 (standard error = 4.7-6.3 beats/min) across low and high intensities of cycle ergometry, treadmill exercise, and bench stepping (Leger & Thivierge, 1988). The conversion of heart rate data to energy expenditure values is based on the linear relationship between heart rate and $\dot{V}O_2$ observed in laboratory tests. A linear regression equation is developed from exercise test data to estimate oxygen consumption, and these values are converted to energy expenditure units (roughly l L of oxygen consumption is equivalent to 5 Kcal of energy expenditure).

Although correlations between heart rate and $\dot{V}O_2$ may be high for an individual exercise test, two regression lines determined for the same individual on different days may show large differences in absolute errors and in the change of errors across the full ranges of heart rate and $\dot{V}O_2$ during physical exertion. For example one study using heart rate to predict oxygen consumption found that the total estimate of energy expenditure during a day was so low (<500 Kcal/d) that use of the heart rate and oxygen consumption relationship obtained during lab testing was meaningless for predicting energy expenditure from heart rates during normal living in 4 of the 17 adults observed (Christensen et al., 1983).

Many investigators have chosen not to follow the recommendation of Booyens and Hervey (1960) that heart rate–$\dot{V}O_2$ regression equations be derived from heart rate and oxygen consumption data collected during activities similar to those to be monitored during the study period. There is a tendency for the heart rate–energy expenditure line to be curved at the lower end and linear at the higher ranges of energy expenditure. The main problem with this method is that the heart rate–$\dot{V}O_2$ relationship varies because of posture, environmental condition, emotional stress, type of muscle contraction, degree of physical conditioning or training, and fatigue. A modest correlation ($r = 0.68$) observed between HR and $\dot{V}O_2$ during moderate-intensity physical activities among adults is markedly improved after statistical adjustment of variations in age and fitness (i.e., $\dot{V}O_2$peak)(Strath et al., 2000).

Regardless of the way the data are handled, heart rates provide objective data, which can be accurately collected from people of all ages with little interruption or restriction of daily activity (Freedson & Miller, 2000). They can even be used by people on medications for lowering heart rate during exertion, if a maximal exercise test is given to establish the range of heart rate from rest to maximal exertion. Some monitors can be used in the water and can store each heartbeat for a period of several days.

Physiological Surrogates

It is known that the amount and rate of physical activity influences maximal oxygen consumption ($\dot{V}O_2$peak); therefore, $\dot{V}O_2$peak has been used as an estimate of physical activity. There are limits to its use as a surrogate measure of physical activity, however. Among adults, about 30 percent of the variation in $\dot{V}O_2$peak is explainable by genetic variation (Perusse et al., 1989). Also, it is not feasible to obtain maximal effort among many people, so it can be difficult to separate the effects of learning and motivation to perform from actual fitness. Moreover, a relatively small portion of the population participates in the type, intensity, and frequency of physical activity sufficient to increase $\dot{V}O_2$peak. Resistance activities (e.g., weightlifting) expend energy and increase strength but do not increase $\dot{V}O_2$peak. Finally, $\dot{V}O_2$peak tends to decrease among boys and girls from age 14 to 18. That decline cannot be explained wholly by physical activity levels, and can partly be accounted for by maturation, especially increased fatness in girls. For these reasons, many experts have felt that $\dot{V}O_2$peak is probably best used in combination with other physical activity estimates or as an indicator of high-intensity activity performed by adults.

Nonetheless, investigators have found a significant relationship between direct and indirect measures of $\dot{V}O_2$peak and self-reported measures of physical activity and dietary estimates of physical activity among adults. Among participants at the Cooper Institute for Aerobics Research in Dallas, for example, correlations between $\dot{V}O_2$peak and a seven-day recall of physical activity have ranged from 0.66 to 0.71 among men and 0.78 to 0.83 among women (Paffenbarger, Blair, Lee, & Hyde, 1993). Other investigators have reported correlations averaging about 0.50 (range from 0.30 to 0.63) between $\dot{V}O_2$peak and several commonly used self-reports of leisure-time physical activity among men and women age 20 to 59 years (Jacobs, Ainsworth, Hartman, & Leon, 1993).

Motion Sensors

Motion sensors to measure physical activity have essentially become movement counters. They provide another objective measure of physical activity that can complement biological markers of physical activity and provide a criterion for judging the validity of self-report of physical activity. Movement counters differ widely in their methodology and accuracy.

Pedometers

Older gear-driven mechanical pedometers have poor reliability and validity as step counters even under highly controlled laboratory conditions (Gayle, Montoye, & Philpot, 1977; Washburn, Chin, & Montoye, 1980). However research on the reliability and validity of newer electronic pedometers, such as the Digi-Walker (Yamax Inc., Tokyo, Japan), is more encouraging. For example Bassett and colleagues (1996) have shown that the Digi-Walker records 100.7 percent (left) and 100.6 percent (right) of steps taken during outdoor walking in 20 adult volunteers. Similarly, Welk and colleagues (2000), in 31 adult volunteers, have shown that the mean step counts from the Digi-Walker during both walking and running on a treadmill and a track were within 3 to 5 percent of the actual values. However, in the same sample, Welk and colleagues reported a rather low correlation ($r = 0.34$) between the average daily step count over a one-week period and average daily energy expenditure assessed by the Stanford Seven-Day Activity Recall. When participants removed the Digi-Walker during all structured vigorous and moderate physical activity, the correlation between the step counts and energy expenditure were near zero ($r = -0.07$). In general, there are some concerns about the interunit reliability of these devices. Also, currently available pedometers do not have a time base or data storage capacity; thus, participants must record numbers from the devices at the beginning and end of the day. It has been suggested that pedometers may serve as a useful criterion measure for validating self-report estimates of walking and as motivational devices for interventions designed to increase walking.

Portable Accelerometers

Although pedometers are simply event counters, portable accelerometers, designed to be worn on a belt at the waist, provide a measure of both frequency and intensity of movement. Currently available portable accelerometers have the advantage of collecting and storing data sequentially over time so that the pattern of physical activity over a day or a number of days can be assessed. The disadvantages to these devices include cost, approximately $300 to $500 per unit, as well as the fact that they are not suitable for aquatic activities, and they do not respond to static activity or activities where there is minimal movement of the body's center of gravity such as rowing or cycling. Within these limitations, portable accelerometers have been a useful addition to the physical activity assessment methodology.

The development of portable accelerometers as physical activity assessment devices was prompted by the observation from laboratory studies conducted in the late 1950s that suggested an association between the integral of vertical acceleration versus time and energy expenditure (Brouha & Smith, 1958; Montoye, Servais, & Webster, 1986). Montoye and colleagues at the University of Wisconsin at Madison were the first to use this principle to develop the prototype for what would later become a commercially available portable accelerometer marketed under the name Caltrac. The Caltrac, like most portable accelerometers, uses a piezoelectric bender element, made of two layers of piezoceramic material with a brass center layer. When the body accelerates, the transducer, mounted on a cantilevered beam, bends, producing an electric charge proportional to the force exerted. An internal computer chip integrates the area under the acceleration and deceleration curve over a defined time interval, stores that value in a computer memory, and resets the integrator.

The Caltrac, unlike the newer generation of portable accelerometers, does not store data in a time sequence but only provides a total estimate of physical activity. A number of studies, in both laboratory and field settings, have shown significant associations between Caltrac readings and energy expenditure measured by indirect calorimetry during walking and running on level surfaces ($r = 0.68\text{-}0.94$) and with energy expenditure during daily activities measured by doubly labeled water over a seven-day period. The lack of data-storage capability, the rather large size, and the poor quality control in manufacturing have led researchers away from using the Caltrac to more sophisticated instruments, such as the Computer Science and Applications (CSA) Actigraph and Biotrainer and TriTrac portable accelerometers.

The CSA Model 7164 portable accelerometer is a small (5.1 cm × 3.8 cm × 1.5 cm, 43 g), single-plane, portable accelerometer that uses a piezoelectric bender element. It is now marketed as Actigraph and distributed by MTI Health Services (Fort Walton Beach, FL). The Actigraph accelerometer is initialized and the data are downloaded using an optical interface connected to the serial port of a personal computer. The investigator can set the start time and data collection interval. The Actigraph has the capacity to store minute-by-minute data for up to 91 days. The downloaded data can be exported to software programs for analysis.

Studies have indicated moderate associations between Actigraph counts per minute and energy expenditure measured by indirect calorimetry during both treadmill and overground walking and running at increasing speeds ($r = 0.66$-0.82) (Hendelman et al., 2000; Melanson & Freedson 1995). However, like all portable accelerometers, counts per minute are not associated with increases in energy cost of locomotion caused by increased grade. The association between Actigraph readings and energy expenditure during other types of physical activity such as house cleaning, golf, and yard work are lower ($r = 0.59$) (Hendelman et al., 2000; Welk et al., 2000).

The Biotrainer (IM Systems, Baltimore, MD) is a single-plane accelerometer similar in size to the Actigraph. The TriTrac (Reining International, Madison, WI) is a three-plane accelerometer, which is considerably larger (170 g) compared with the others. Welk and colleagues (2000) compared Actigraph, Biotrainer, and TriTrac output in 52 adults who completed two 30-minute activity scenarios including treadmill walking or jogging and simulated "lifestyle" activities with energy expenditure measured by indirect calorimetry. Results indicated that the correlation between accelerometer readings and energy expenditure were higher during treadmill activity (mean $r = 0.86$) compared with lifestyle activities (mean $r = 0.55$). Correlations between the Actigraph, Biotrainer, and TriTrac were high during both treadmill ($r = 0.86$) and lifestyle activity ($r = 0.70$), suggesting that similar information is obtained from all three accelerometers. In theory, the use of a multiplane accelerometer would provide a better estimate of body movement and thus energy expenditure. However, recent studies (e.g., Welk et al., 2000; Hendelman et al., 2000) have shown little advantage to using the larger and more complex three-plane accelerometer (TriTrac) over the smaller and less complex single-plane accelerometers.

In the future, the use of motion sensors in population-based research will most likely increase. As the price of this technology declines, the feasibility of monitoring a large number of individuals over several days will increase. In the meantime, the portable accelerometer will continue to be a useful criterion measure for the validation of self-report physical activity assessment instruments. To provide a better understanding of the dose-response relationship between physical activity intensity and chronic disease risk, it is important that better self-report measures of physical activity intensity be developed. Heart rate monitoring and portable accelerometers have been suggested as criteria for assessing the intensity of daily physical activity. Several investigators have attempted to define cut points for accelerometer counts per minute that correspond to various MET levels of activity; however, the results of these studies have not been encouraging. For example, three reports have shown that the cut point for Actigraph counts per minute for activity of three METs or greater vary by tenfold. Further work is needed in order to more clearly define these cut points for activity intensity and to clearly delineate the physical activity dimensions for which the cut points are valid, especially among frail elderly people whose vertical accelerations of mass during physical activity may be markedly reduced compared to young and middle-aged people.

Simultaneous monitoring of heart rate and motion counts provides corroborating estimates of physical activity that can agree highly in some people under controlled conditions or can provide independent and additive estimates of physical activity among different people in more diverse settings. Haskell and colleagues (1993) have shown that the use of individual HR–$\dot{V}O_2$ slopes in addition to arm- and leg-motion sensors in a linear regression model yielded a multiple correlation squared of 0.89 with a standard error of 2.3 ml · kg · min^{-1} during walking, running, arm cranking, cycling, and bench stepping.

Specific Features of Physical Activity

The measurement of specific features of physical activity is important for at least two reasons. First, understanding the biological explanations for why physical activity may protect against specific diseases that have different causes requires that physiological adaptations to physical activity be determined, such as shown in table 6.2. Such physiological adaptations will differ according to the types, amounts, and rates of physical activity (Pollock et al., 1998). Thus, it is necessary that specific features of physical activity be measured. Similarly, determining whether different dose-response relationships exist between physical activity and different diseases also requires that specifics about physical activity be assessed.

Second, understanding people's motivation to be physically active also requires measures of physical activity specifics because people may differ according to their willingness to engage in physical activities that differ in type, frequency, duration, and intensity. The weak to moderate agreement among different measures of physical activity presents a special problem in this regard (Dishman, 1994). For example, we reported that the relationship between social-cognitive variables and self-reported free-living

Table 6.2   Specific Features and Measures of Physical Activity Hypothetically Related to Disease Outcomes

Feature	Mechanism	Measure	Disease outcome
Calorie	Energy cost	Doubly labeled H$_2$O	Heart disease, type 2 diabetes, obesity, cancer
Aerobic intensity	Cardiac function	Oxygen uptake	Heart disease, type 2 diabetes
Weight bearing or loading	Gravity or force	Motion sensor	Osteoporosis
Flexibility	ROM	Goniometer	Disability
Muscular strength	Force	Dynamometer	Disability

ROM = range of motion.

Adapted from Caspersen 1989.

physical activity did not generalize to physical activity estimated by the Caltrac accelerometer (Dishman, Darracott, & Lambert, 1992).

It may be helpful to conceptualize physical activity as a latent construct and use methods such as structural equation modeling and latent growth curve modeling, as illustrated in figure 6.5, in large sample studies to determine the relative contributions of the available physical activity measures to the construct of physical activity and its change. Such approaches can also be used to examine whether the composite physical activity score or its components are more closely related to the determinants and health-related outcomes of physical activity among older people.

It will be important to consider limitations of available measures that might be exaggerated among older people (see table 6.3), especially people who have age-associated disabilities that affect gait, memory, or metabolism in ways that can influence the relationships between features of physical activity or energy expenditure and existing measures.

Conclusion

No single method of physical activity assessment fully meets the criteria of being reliable, valid, practical, and noninterfering with usual activity (see table 6.1). Even the highly valid and increasingly practical method of doubly labeled water used to estimate energy expenditure does not provide information about dimensions of physical activity such as intensity, mode, frequency, and social context and other behavioral components such as timing. At present, the standard errors of estimating energy expenditure by linear regression of $\dot{V}O_2$ on heart rate or accelerometer counts range

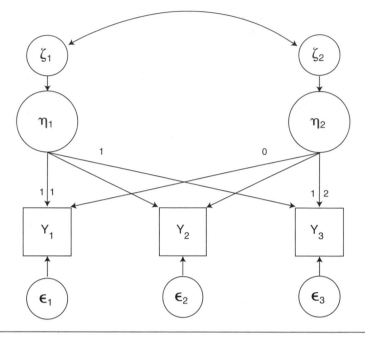

Figure 6.5 Latent growth modeling of change in physical activity measured as a latent variable. η_1 is initial status. η_2 is change function. Y_1-Y_3 indicates physical activity measured three times. Initial status (01); change function (02); linear (0,1,2), quadratic (1,2,4), unspecified (0,1,L); ζ = disturbance term, i.e., unexplained variance; ϵ = uniqueness, i.e., error.

Table 6.3   Measurement Issues for Older People

	Issue?	Nonissue?
Accuracy of recall		*
Types of physical activity	*	

Motion sensors
  Gain (force vs. mass displacement)
  Fat-free mass vs. EE/RMR
	*	*

Biological markers
  HR vs. $\dot{V}O_2$
  Doubly labeled H_2O
		*
		*

EE = energy expenditure; RMR = resting metabolic rate.

from about 5 to 25 percent during activities that involve locomotion. Each of the popular methods for physical activity assessment (self-report, calorimetry, doubly labeled water, heart rate monitoring, fitness change, and accelerometry) is sufficiently accurate to classify individuals according to tertiles or quartiles of energy expenditure without the risk of high levels of misclassification. This degree of precision is adequate to permit determination of whether most determinants or health-related outcomes are related to physical activity in a linear or quadratic pattern when a group of several hundred people is studied. Using scores obtained using these methods to rank individuals within small groups (e.g., less than 100) will undoubtedly result in substantial errors when estimating their true activity levels or energy expenditure resulting from physical activity.

Physical activity is a multidimensional behavior such that no single assessment method or tool can capture all its dimensions. The method chosen to assess physical activity must depend on the research problem being addressed and the constraints imposed by sample size, time, setting, and budget. To obtain a more global estimate of physical activity, multiple assessment methods should be utilized. The use of multiple methods can contribute to the understanding of the relations among different techniques.

CHAPTER 7

Assessing Physical Performance in Older Adults

M. Elaine Cress, PhD

The prevalence of dependency in activities of daily living escalates from 7 percent for people 65 to 74 years of age to greater than 24 percent for those over 84 years of age (Guralnik & Simonsick, 1993). Accommodation of the changes of aging in order to live independently depends on the balance and reserve in physical and cognitive abilities.

When Mrs. Barkley, age 88, is asked to identify those things that are most important to her quality of life, she quickly replies her home and her dog. She lives in the same home where she raised her three children and continues to volunteer as a librarian. Tending to her three-bedroom home requires a fairly active schedule of watering the lawn and daily feedings for her dog, the birds, and the squirrels. She is generally in good health; however, she experiences shortness of breath upon exertion, which is unresponsive to the inhalant medication prescribed by her doctor. She is motivated to participate in strength training two days per week because she believes it will help her maintain her independence. Because driving is an essential skill for her independent lifestyle, she has decreased her exposure to accidents by curtailing her driving at sunset and out of her hometown. A couple of times a year, Mrs. Barkley travels out of the country alone or with her sister, age 92, and her brother, age 84. These excursions require that she make considerable arrangements, including having her passport and caring for her dog. Mrs. Barkley relies heavily on her cognitive ability to sustain her quality of life. She manages her deteriorating physical abilities by minimizing the trips to the grocery store, managing her medication, and getting help from a reliable social network. Through good judgment she has avoided automobile accidents and falls.

The Nagi sociomedical model of disablement is a heuristic model for organizing interrelated components of pathology impairment, functional limitation, and disability (Nagi, 1976, 1991). This model (Nagi, 1991) describes a single pathway with progressive deterioration from cellular pathology to whole-person disability. In the Nagi model, pathology is an identified injury or disease process that leads to an impairment of an organ system such as the musculoskeletal, neurological, cardiovascular, or pulmonary systems. Impairments are directly linked to functional limitation in such activities as bathing, dressing, toileting, and basic mobility. Disability is the ultimate outcome where an individual can no longer maintain his or her role in society.

Evidence of the causal ordering of this pathway was provided in a longitudinal study by Lawrence and Jette (1996) in which predisposing factors, pathology, and impairments are direct predictors of functional limitation and indirectly predict disability. Functional capacity can be defined as an individual's inherent capability to perform fundamental physical, emotional, or mental actions (Verbrugge & Jette, 1994). Although the Nagi model is useful in linking single pathology to disability, 30 percent of people over 65 have three or more chronic conditions. The confluence of multiple system declines that lead to functional limitation and disability has been called a *geriatric syndrome* (Reuben, 1991).

Geriatric syndrome can be illustrated using the various scenarios listed in table 7.1. Table 7.1 demonstrates how cognitive performance, physical

Table 7.1   Nagi Model of Disablement With Specific, Noncomprehensive Examples

Pathology	Impairment	Functional limitation	Disability
Cognitive			
	Memory	Inability to plan Forget to get medications	No passport for the trip Trip is delayed while medication is ordered.
	Processing speed	Driving: failure to change course quickly (e.g., getting on the freeway in a timely fashion)	Everything takes longer so there may be a failure to get the basic living chores done each day.
	Slow reaction time	Failure to move quickly to alter the course	Must use another exit May result in an accident
Physical			
Sarcopenia	Weak muscles	Inability to carry a large suitcase	Require help or use a smaller suitcase
	Low muscle power	Inability to move quickly	May not be able to move quickly enough to stop a fall
	Slow reaction time	Low function	

performance, and motor processing may interact to impair Mrs. Barkley's ability to function independently. High cognitive functioning can ameliorate the impact of physical disability. For example, consider the case of noted physicist Stephen Hawking. He has done most of his work, including authoring his 1988 book, *A Brief History of Time*, after the onset of the progressive neurological disease amyotrophic lateral sclerosis. Many older adults can function successfully into their later years in spite of declining physical health.

Conversely, although impairment as a result of chronic disease explains approximately 80 percent of disabilities, epidemiological studies indicate that up to 20 percent of disablement is in the absence of up to 15 of the most common chronic conditions as reported by Femia, Zarit, and Johansson (2001). This revealing statistic prompted a further investigation of the role of psychosocial factors such as depression, cognitive status, subjective health, and social integration in explaining disability in the oldest old of the Swedish Twins Study (Femia, Zarit, & Johansson, 2001). In this population-based study, a sample of 351 twin pairs, 85 years of age and older were tested at three levels on the disablement model: impairment, functional limitations, and disability. Risk factors such as age and socioeconomic status, as well as psychosocial factors and internal resources such as depression, locus of control, emotion, and vigor were also assessed. A series of structural models on the data were constructed to evaluate the main pathway of disability and a full model of disability that included risk factors and psychosocial variables. Being 85 was associated with greater impairments, lower ratings of subjective health, less social isolation, and greater disability. Grip strength was a robust predictor of disability and retained a direct relationship to disability even when psychosocial variables were controlled. Grip strength directly predicted disability as well as being mediated by cognition. In addition, grip strength predicted both upper- and lower-body functional limitations in the main Nagi pathway as illustrated in table 7.1. Grip strength has a consistently strong and direct relationship to disability, indicating the power of the variable to predict disability.

Visual impairment had significant direct effects on lower-body function limitations, but these influences were shifted to upper-body functional limitations after accounting for psychosocial variables. Furthermore, visual impairment had direct effects on subjective health and depression. Cognitive impairment and depression were bidirectional. The authors explained that preexisting dementia with depression would not hasten disability; however, depression with the addition of dementia could strongly accelerate disability. A physical impairment, such as limited vision, exacerbates depressive symptomology, which in turn is related to poorer cognitive status. Social isolation is highly correlated with more depression and lower subjective health. Moreover, upper- and lower-body functional limitations were related to social isolation, a mediator of disability along with depression

(Femia et al., 2001). The primary importance of this study is its identification of the role of psychosocial factors in nearly one-quarter of the population sample with disability in the absence of physical impairment. In particular, depression was identified as an important mediating factor that could be a warning sign of vulnerability to impending disablement.

Several mediators of physical dependency, including depression, are responsive to exercise training. Using a meta-analysis of the literature, North, McCullagh, and Tran (1990) found that endurance training was as effective as psychotherapy in reducing depression. Combined endurance and strength training are effective interventions for increasing upper- and lower-body function (Cress et al., 1999). In a randomized controlled trial of men and women 70 years old or older, who were without disability but who were shifting from highly independent living arrangements to an apartment or retirement community, engaged in six months of exercise or usual activity (control). The exercise group improved its ability to perform common daily tasks by 14 percent with an effect size of 0.94. Significant improvement in the domains of upper- and lower-body strength and endurance all contributed to the overall improvement in physical functional performance. At baseline, the control and exercise groups that had similar physical functional performance scores on the Continuous-Scale Physical Functional Performance (CS-PFP) Test (CS-PFP: 55.3 ± 14 and 54.3 ± 14, respectively) were at the threshold of independence (57 CS-PFP units) (Cress & Meyers, 2003), as identified in subsequent work by the same team. Any loss in fitness (strength or aerobic capacity) results in a much greater loss in function for people below the threshold of 57 CS-PFP units than for those above the threshold. Those having a CS-PFP score of higher than 57 enjoy a physical reserve that can act as a buffer against functional decline. Following the intervention, the exercise group had a CS-PFP score of 62.1 ± 15, providing substantial physical reserve. Thus, rather than viewing these individuals as having functional limitation, the concept of physical reserve captures a notion of functional ability or even resilience.

Recently, efforts have been made to reframe the language from that of "disablement" to "enablement" and from that of "functional limitation" to "functional ability" (Brandt & Pope, 1997). Mrs. Barkley's quality of life and ability to live independently is defined in relation to the demand placed on her by her home. Verbrugge and Jette (1994) expanded the main pathway developed by the Nagi (1991) model to include environmental demand and personal ability as contextual terms for defining *disability*. For example, if two people have the same functional limitation—the inability to climb a flight of stairs—and one person lives in a second-floor apartment and the other lives on the first floor, the one who has to overcome the environmental demand has a disability, whereas the person living on the first floor does not. This example illustrates the notion of disability as a reflection of a gap between a person's ability and the context of environmental demand (Brandt & Pope, 1997; Verbrugge & Jette, 1994).

This view of physical disability as the balance between physical capability and environmental demand is similar to the "environmental-press" model put forth by Lawton and Nahemow (1973). The environmental-press model seeks to explain the range of behavioral patterns, such as frustration and confidence, within the context of environmental demand and personal competency in mental, emotional, and physical domains. Psychological factors are internal resources that enable a person to cope, adapt, control, and manipulate the environment successfully to prolong independence. More internal resources can compensate for functional limitation in the physical domain and having less can aggravate it (Femia et al., 2001). The reasoning is that greater cognitive ability allows a person to respond and adapt to the demands of the environment and remain engaged at a higher level of functioning (Femia et al., 2001).

Dementia and lower cognitive performance are independent risk factors (Femia et al., 2001; Gill, Richardson, & Tinetti, 1995), while persons with greater depression or neuroticism are more apt to report disability (Jang et al., 2002) in the absence of a physical impairment. Depression and poor performance on cognitive assessment are predictive of greater change in disability (Femia et al., 2001). Depression hampers the motivation to make appropriate lifestyle changes necessary for sustaining an independent lifestyle, and therefore it leads to a faster slide into disability (Femia et al., 2001). Depression, however, may affect self-reported measures of function more than objective performance (Cress et al., 1995). A depressed person may overreport functional limitation, feeling the impending danger to his or her health because of illness. The ability to accommodate and adapt has been shown to be mediated by depression, subjective health, and social integration (Femia et al., 2001). Planning interventions, such as physical activity, that address these mediators are as important as strategies to address primary mental and physical limitations.

This chapter focuses on the scientific literature that addresses the following:

1. Methods of assessing physical functional performance in older adults

2. Relationship of measures of cognitive performance to measures of functional performance and disability

3. Contribution of cognitive performance and lower-extremity impairment to physical performance

4. Evidence for physical training to alter directly the course of functional limitation and disability

5. Recommendations for future directions in research

Assessment of Physical Function in Older Adults

Changes in life expectancy have resulted in a dramatic increase in the elderly population. Through the life course for those individuals who become disabled, there is a transitioning from good health and high functioning to poor health or disability or both. For primary and secondary prevention of disability it is necessary to adequately screen, assess, and objectively measure physical function for purposes that range from public policy to personal planning. The progression of functional decline within the axes of declining health and advancing age is described in figure 7.1.

Depending on the stage of health and age (see figure 7.1), different functional measures are needed in order to discriminate functional status and to detect the change in status. The two primary assessment techniques include questionnaire-based measures of self-reported function and objective or performance-based measures of functional tasks.

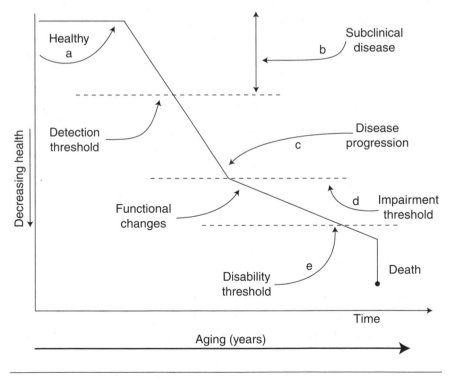

Figure 7.1 Opportunities for prevention.

These two measures have been shown to be moderately correlated (r = –0.194 to –0.625) when using self-reported and performance-based measures of ambulation (Cress et al., 1995). In the presence of clinical depression or cognitive impairment, performance-based measures of function provide a more reliable and accurate assessment of an individual's physical function (Cress et al., 1995; Mahurin, DeBettignies, & Pirozzolo, 1991).

Instrument characteristics are important considerations when choosing a functional assessment tool. Test–retest reproducibility, validity, and sensitivity to change (Buchner, Guralnik, & Cress, 1995) are fundamental considerations in choosing an instrument. A valid assessment evaluates the characteristic it is intended to measure. A reliable instrument can be administered with reproducible results from day to day and among trained administrators. Instrument sensitivity is the ability of the assessment to detect meaningful change over time.

In general, clinical measures of function can easily be performed by people who are healthy (figure 7.1 segment *a*) or who have subclinical disease (figure 7.1 segment *b*). For example, highly functioning individuals are able to stand for 10 seconds in tandem heel-to-toe. Ability to detect change is compromised because receiving the highest score at baseline cannot detect improvement caused by an intervention. This measurement anomaly is known as a "ceiling effect." On the other hand, if a measure is comprised of tasks that very few older adults are able to accomplish, it said to have a "floor effect." For example, a person unable to rise from a chair without using the hands to push off from the chair will score a zero on a test that requires standing from a chair without using the arms. None of the performance measures that include chair stands as a timed task allow the use of hands (e.g., National Institute on Aging (NIA) short performance battery, Fullerton Fitness Test). If the person improves but still cannot stand without the aid of the arms, the score will still reflect a zero, minimizing the ability to detect change. Instruments with ceiling or floor effects can be used to assess only a narrow range of physical ability. Because of the narrow range of detection, improvement or decline must be in that range in order for change to be detected. Another factor that minimizes an instrument's sensitivity to change is the graduation of the scaling. Some performance-based measures group the range of performance into quartiles of the population, giving the lowest performance a score of one and the highest performance a score of four (e.g., NIA short performance battery, Physical Performance Test). Any change in performance that is within the grouping will go undetected. For example, walking eight feet at normal pace in 5.5 seconds prior to an intervention that improves to 4.6 seconds after an intervention yields the same score of two on the NIA short performance battery (Guralnik et al., 1994). The functional levels of the population (figure 7.1), as well as the scaling of the instrument are both important considerations when identifying the most appropriate assessment measure for a given population.

Several performance-based tests are listed in table 7.2. This is not intended as an exhaustive list, but rather we have restricted it to those tests commonly used for research and possibly in a clinical setting. These tests are organized into categories based on the population that can be most appropriately assessed considering the ceiling and floor effects of the tests. The categories include (1) nonambulatory (figure 7.1 segment *e*), (2) balance and low functioning but ambulatory (figure 7.1, segment *d*), and (3) moderate- to high-functioning mobility (figure 7.1, segments *b* and *c*). Performance-based measures with tasks appropriate for assessment of function in people who are nonambulatory include the Physical Performance and Mobility Exam (Winograd et al., 1994) and the Physical Disability Index (Gerety et al., 1993). Assessments of balance include the Frailty and Injuries: Cooperative Studies of Intervention Techniques (FICSIT) balance measure (Rossitier-Fornoff, Wolf, Wolfson, & Buchner, 1995), the functional reach test (Duncan, Weiner, Chandler, & Studenski, 1990), and the Tinetti Performance-Oriented Mobility Scale (Tinetti, 1986). Assessments that are appropriate for mobile and highly functioning individuals can be divided into single-task tests or those without summary scores and multiple-task tests with summary scores. Multiple-task measures that do not have a summary score and single-task measures may be less sensitive to detecting change than multiple tasks with a summary score. Single-task tests or those without summary scores include usual gait (Buchner et al., 1995), the Timed Up and Go Test (Podsiadlo & Richardson, 1991), and the Fullerton Fitness Test (Rikli & Jones, 1999). Multiple-task tests that have summary scores include the short performance-based battery from the Study of Established Populations Epidemiological Studies (Guralnik et al., 1994), the Physical Performance Test (Reuben, Siu, & Kimpau, 1992), and the Continuous-Scale Physical Functional Performance Test (Cress et al., 1996). The tests are summarized in table 7.2.

Each of these tests has been validated on populations between healthy (figure 7.1 segment *a*) and individuals with disabilities (figure 7.1 segment *e*). Validation research uses a cross-sectional design in order to assess a broad range of individuals (Cress et al., 1996; Duncan et al., 1990; Reuben et al., 1992; Winograd et al., 1994; Guralnik et al., 1994; Gerety et al., 1993). Common tasks that have distinct end points are the most reliably administered tasks (Jette, Jette, et al., 1999). Test–retest reliability is dependent on several factors including (1) distinct starting and end points for the timing of the tasks (Jette, Jette, et al., 1999; Cress et al., 1996); (2) standardized dialogue used for administration of the test (Cress et al., 1996); (3) commonality of the tasks that are administered (for example, walking at usual pace is common, whereas rising from a chair with the arms folded across the chest is not a common functional task) (Jette, Jette, et al., 1999); and (4) muscular and functional limitations that introduce test–retest variability. People with chronic disability conditions (figure 7.1 segments *d* and *e*) such as rheumatoid or osteoarthritis have greater day-to-day performance variation. Thus, for individuals that are the most difficult to study, a larger number of subjects is needed to detect change. Detection of small differences generated by interventions, however, depends not only on the strength of the intervention but also on how well the instrument (see table 7.2) is matched to the stage of functional status of the population (see figure 7.1). Instruments that are well suited for assessing function in populations that are at or below the threshold of disability (line *e* and below on figure 7.1) include the Physical Performance Mobility Exam (Winograd et al., 1994) and the Physical Disability Index (Gerety, 1993) (table 7.2). These measures have been used to assess function in those with severe mobility impairments and include hospitalized patients and residents of skilled nursing care facilities, respectively. Between the impairment (line *d*) and the disability threshold (line *e*) is a stage of rapid functional change. Balance measures such as the Performance-Oriented Mobility Scale (Tinetti, 1986), functional reach test (Duncan et al., 1990), and the FICSIT balance scale (Rossitier-Fornoff et al., 1995) are effective assessment tools in this stage. Measures of the Fullerton Fitness Test (Rikli & Jones, 1999), Physical Performance Test (Reuben et al., 1992), Continuous-Scale Physical Functional Performance Test (CS-PFP) (Cress et al., 1996), Timed Up and Go Test (Podsiadlo & Richardson, 1991), and the NIA short performance battery (Guralnik et al., 1994) have been shown to assess function in this stage (lines *d-e*).

To prevent disability, steps have been taken to identify preclinical disability (Fried et al., 1997) and risk factors for functional decline (Fried et al., 1991). The CS-PFP is an instrument useful for detecting functional change that develops during the progression of disease (figure 1, segment *c*). Consider cardiovascular disease, an example of geriatric syndromes, where the disease silently develops in several systems eroding health and physical reserves well before a person notices a decline in function. Until the disease affects daily functioning or because of overt denial, *self-reported* functional measures fail to show any functional limitation. Most of the performance measures reported in table 7.2 fail to detect the impending deficits. The CS-PFP can detect changes in function prior to an overt awareness of functional change, and, in addition, the domain scores of function (strength, endurance, and balance and coordination) have been shown to identify change in individuals in experiencing the stage of disease progression (figure 7.1 line *c*) (Brochu et al., 2002; Cress et al., 1999; Miszko et al., 2003). The functional threshold (57 CS-PFP units) discussed earlier is associated with physical thresholds of aerobic peak performance

Table 7.2   Performance-Based Measures of Physical Function and Selected Measurement Characteristics

Test name	Tasks	Metric	Scaling	Summary scores
Nonambulatory				
Physical Performance Mobility Exam (PPME) (Winograd et al. 1994)	Bed mobility[1] Chair transfer Sit-to-stand Balance stances[2]	Time	0-6 0-12 Pass/fail	Yes 0-6 or 0-12
Physical Disability Index (PDI) (Gerety et al., 1993)	Bed mobility Chair transfer Sit-to-stand Balance stances 180° or 360° turn Gait speed or distance	Time ROM Weight (kg)	Continuous	No
Ambulatory				
Usual gait (Buchner et al., 1995)	Walking	Time (s)	Continuous	No
Functional reach (Duncan et al. 1990)	Forward reach in stance	Inches	Continuous	No
Tinetti Performance-Oriented Mobility Scale (Tinetti et al., 1986)	Sitting balance Chair transfer Sit-to-stand Comfortable stance Sternal push Turn Gait speed Gait parameters[3]	Time Distance	Continuous	
FICSIT balance	Balance stances[2]	Time (s)	Ordinal	No

Floor	Ceiling	Sensitivity to change	Time to complete	Administrative requirements and considerations
Insufficient studies to comment	Insufficient studies to comment	No published data found	< 15 min	• Requires a step • Requires a bed with handrail • Easy to administer • No extensive training required
Insufficient studies to comment	Insufficient studies to comment	No published data found (Gerety et al., 1993)	45 min to 1 h	None
No	Yes, if baseline gait is >1 m/s (Buchner et al., 1996)	Yes, if < 1 m/s at baseline (Buchner et al., 1996)	< 5 min	Requires a space > 6 m
No	Yes, in populations without balance impairments	No (Morey et al., 1999) Yes, in those needing rehabilitation (Weiner et al., 1993)	< 5 min	Requires a ruler
No	Yes, in populations without balance impairments	Effect size = 1.7 (Tinetti et al., 1999)	< 15 min	None
Yes	$ES = 0.16$ (Tinetti et al., 1999)		< 15 min	None

(continued)

Table 7.2   *(continued)*

Test name	Tasks	Metric	Scaling	Summary scores
Ambulatory tests with no summary scale or single-task tests				
Timed Up and Go (Podsiadlo & Richardson, 1991)	Gait speed	Overall score in time	Continuous	Single task
Fullerton Fitness	Arm curl[4] Chair stand[4] Sit and reach Shoulder flex (back stretch) 6-min walk 8-ft Up and Go	Number of repetitions in 30 s, time, distance	Continuous	No
Ambulatory tests with a summary score				
National Institute on Aging short performance battery (Guralnik et al., 1994)	Balance stances[2] 5-chair stand repetitions Gait speed	Time (s)	Ordinal 1-4 for each task Total score 0-12	Yes
Continuous Scale-Physical Functional Performance Test (Cress et al., 1996)	Upper-body strength[5] Upper-body flexibility[6] Lower-body strength[7] Balance and coordination[8], and endurance[9]	Time Distance Weight	Continuous 1-100	Yes

124

Floor	Ceiling	Sensitivity to change	Time to complete	Administrative requirements and considerations
No, if ambulatory	In high-functioning populations scoring ≤5 s	$ES = 0.09$ (Jette et al., 1999) No, insufficient data to calculate effect size (Ouellet & Moffett, 2002)	<5 min	Requires a chair and stopwatch
On specific tasks (e.g., arm curl, chair stand, 8 ft [2.4 m] Up and Go)	On specific tasks (e.g., arm curl, 8 ft [2.4 m] Up and Go)	No effect size data published	15-30 min	Requires 5 (2.3 kg) and 8 lb (3.6 kg) weights Chair Walking space ≥ 80 m
On chair stand ambulation	Yes, if no impairment or limitation	Data for effect size not available (Reuben et al., 1999; Hausdorff et al., 2001; Ostir, Markides, Black, & Goodwin, 1998)	<15 min	Chair >2.4 m (8 ft) area
Yes for floor sit-to-stand (Cress et al., 1996)	None found (Cress & Meyer, 2003)	$ES = 0.7$ (Cress et al., 1999)	30-60 min	Requires area ≥213 m (700 ft) Hallway 91 m (300 ft) Stairs Weights Pots Washer/dryer Groceries Carrying bags Bed Jacket Scarves Requirements can be found at www.coe.uga.edu/cs-pfp

(continued)

Table 7.2   *(continued)*

Test name	Tasks	Metric	Scaling	Summary scores
Ambulatory tests with a summary score *(continued)*				
Physical Performance Test (Reuben et al., 1992)	Pick up object from floor Climb stairs Put book on shelf Write a sentence Feeding Gait speed	Time (s)	Ordinal 0-24 0-36	Yes

1. Movements in bed: supine to sit, sit

2. Balance stances: comfortable stance, parallel stance, semitandem stance, tandem stance

3. Gait parameters: gait initiation, step frequency, step length and stride length, walking base, step height, step symmetry, step continuity, trunk stability, walk stance

4. Number of repetitions in 30 s

5. Upper-body strength domain: carry and pour water, carry weight, transfer laundry, sweep, grocery carry weight, time to open fire door

(20 ml · kg^{-1} · min^{-1}) and knee extensor strength (2.5 N · m/kg · m^{-1}) (Cress & Meyer, 2003). Changes assessed using the Cs-PFP provide evidence of change in both function and fitness. Selected single-item measures such as the six-minute walk, which is a part of the Fullerton Fitness and the CS-PFP tests may be sensitive to change for those with preclinical disability. The Physical Performance Test (Reuben et al., 1992) is an example of a measure that has a ceiling effect at baseline when being used on a population that doesn't have functional limitation (figure 7.1 segment *b*) (Binder, Storandt, & Birge, 1999; Papadakis et al., 1996). On the other hand, this measure is sensitive to change when the target population has a preexisting functional limitation (Binder et al., 2002). Having an awareness of functional change during the progression of a disease provides an opportunity to deal with the impact of the disease on the health and functional status of the individual. Cardiovascular diseases also limit blood flow to the brain, leading to the eventual decline in cognitive performance and mental status (See chapters 4 and 9 of this volume.). As illustrated by figure 7.1, physical function does not decline in a linear fashion. How physical and cognitive domains interact to compensate for deficits and preserve functional status is not well understood. Research studies are needed to help delineate these relationships and the optimal interventions for affecting overall function and to provide direction in prevention and treatment of functional decline.

Floor	Ceiling	Sensitivity to change	Time to complete	Administrative requirements and considerations
No published data on floor effects	Yes (Papadakis et al. 1996)	Data to calculate effect size not available. Significant change with exercise in group with functional limitation	15-30 min	Small common items Stairs Hallway 15 m (50 ft)

Upper-body flexibility domain: time to put on and remove a jacket, highest distance reached

Lower-body strength domain: weight carried, sweep time, vacuum time, bed-making time, weight carried onto bus platform, weight of groceries carried, time to climb 11 stairs, time to sit down and rise from the floor, sweep, vacuum

Balance and coordination: time on all timed tasks

Endurance domain: time on all timed tasks and distance covered in 6 min

Contribution of Cognitive Performance and Lower-Extremity Impairment to Physical Performance

Motor processing skills such as reaction time illustrate the essential link between central and peripheral nervous systems in the performance of tasks. Simple response time is made up of central processing for initiation of an action and movement time for task completion, a reflection of the peripheral nervous system. Higher fitness and younger age are associated with shorter reaction times (Spirduso & Clifford, 1978). Reaction time increases by approximately 5 percent per decade beginning around age 30 (Spirduso, 1980). Higher physical performance is associated with quicker movement time when taking a full step forward (Cress et al., 1996). Loss of muscle mass and the association with the reduction in fast-twitch (Type II) muscle fibers with advancing years is well documented (Aniansson, Grimby, Nygaard, & Saltin, 1980). Reduction in the ability to generate force, 7.5 percent to 8.5 percent per decade, parallels the reduction in mass (Larsson, Grimby, & Karlsson, 1979). Power, the generation of force per unit of time, is important for the performance of everyday tasks. Lower-extremity power, as measured using the Nottingham Leg Power Rig

(Nottingham, UK), is associated with faster stair-climbing and walking speed (Bassey et al., 1992,). Lower production of force and slower reaction time combine to amplify the decline in leg-extensor power (LEP) by approximately 35 percent per decade between 60 and 90 years of age (Young & Skelton, 1994). The reduction in LEP is largely due to a reduction in contraction velocity (DeVito et al., 1998). Habitual physical activity and lower-extremity power contribute independently to self-reported physical function and account for 40 percent of the variance in self-reported function (Foldvari et al., 2000; Liemohn, 1975). Those with low levels of LEP have difficulty climbing stairs (Bassey et al., 1992) and may be compromised in recovering from falls (Dutta, Hadley, & Lexell, 1997). Reduced muscle electrical activity (EMG) secondary to a concurrent cognitive task suggests that attentional factors compromise motor control (Rankin et al., 2000). Consider that Mrs. Barkley is crossing a busy city street and pacing her crossing with the crosswalk signal. In addition, she is given a dual task to watch for cars turning into the pedestrian walkway. Her leg power is critical for achieving the necessary walking pace, her attention must be given to risk factors for her safety, and her executive function is needed to assess the time available to cross the street and to govern the pace of her gait. The relationships of these physical and cognitive domains were tested in a broad range of older men and women who lived in the community at large (Petrella, Miller, & Cress, 2004). Volunteers were categorized as independent if little or no functional limitation was reported and as marginally dependent if functional limitation was reported. The Continuous-Scale Physical Functional Performance Test was measured to provide a summary score of physical function from 16 tasks of everyday function such as making a bed, carrying groceries, and sweeping the floor. Lower-extremity power was significantly related to physical function ($r = 0.658$) and to processing speed ($r = 0.408$) (Petrella et al., 2004). CS-PFP was modestly related to reaction time ($r = -0.405$) and significantly related to processing speed ($r = 0.687$). Regression analysis using physical and cognitive models were performed to predict independent living status. In the physical model, both the lower-extremity power and the CS-PFP predicted independent living status in 68 percent of the participants. In the cognitive model, reaction time and memory correctly predicted independent living status for 79 percent of the participants. These cross-sectional data suggest that people with higher cognitive performance to process information quickly (central nervous system) and the ability to generate power to act on those decisions (peripheral) have increased physical function. These two domains explain almost three-quarters of the physical functional performance in older adults. The question remains as to what these correlations mean and how to explain the relationship between exercise and cognition.

Physical Training Interventions

The ability to live independently in later years is one of the highest priorities of older adults. Understanding the underlying determinants of function can provide insight into appropriate interventions for sustaining independence. A large body of scientific publications supports the importance of physical activity to the health and functioning of older adults. Exercise interventions directed toward impairments in cognitive and physical domains have generally been evaluated separately. The effects of physical activity on cognitive status are reviewed in chapters 1 to 3 of this volume. In this section a brief overview of the benefits of exercise regimens on impairments and functional limitations are presented, followed by an exploration of mind and body exercise for improving both cognitive and physical function.

The physical benefits of engaging in late-life exercise are well documented in a comprehensive review (Singh, 2002). Exercise interventions have been effective at several levels on the Nagi model of disablement (Keysor & Jette, 2001). Physical activity is important for prevention and management of pathological conditions (U.S. Department of Health and Human Services, 1996). Many excellent randomized controlled trials have demonstrated that older adults can improve strength 40 to 150 percent and improve endurance (Singh, 2002). In a comprehensive review of the literature, Keysor and Jette (2001) present evidence showing that physical exercise training improves functional limitations. Men and women 70 years old and older can improve their physical performance by approximately 15 percent using a combined endurance and strength training program (Cress et al., 1999) or a power training program (Miszko et al., 2003). Moreover, resistance training may improve physical limitations without changing the underlying pathology.

Thirty older women who had experienced a myocardial infarction at least six months prior to participation in the six-month resistance training program increased their physical functional performance by 24 percent without changing the underlying cardiovascular deficiencies (Brochu et al., 2002). The overwhelming evidence is that physical training improves functional limitations that if left unchecked may lead to disability. Although the evidence for physical training improving disability is less convincing (Keysor & Jette, 2001), strength training has also been effective for improving disability in older adults with osteoarthritis (Ettinger et al., 1997).

Most studies have evaluated exercise training protocols targeting a specific pathology such as cardiovascular disease (Ades, Waldmann, & Gillespie, 1995) or a domain of impairment such as lack of strength (Fiatarone et al., 1994). However, evidence cited earlier in this chapter indicates that combined cognitive and physical impairments result in a fivefold increase in disability over either alone (Gill, Williams, Richardson, & Tinetti, 1996). Perhaps interventions that address both domains could provide the greatest opportunity for functional benefit for time spent in exercise. Mind and body exercise regimens such as yoga from India and tai chi chuan and qigong from China have evolved over many millennia. The goal of these exercise regimens is to manage energy or vital life force, sometimes called *chi*. Only in recent years have Western scientific studies begun to include these exercise protocols in research studies. It is difficult to quantify intensity and standardize the exercise stimulus across individuals in these holistic forms of exercise.

A review by Luskin and colleagues of mind and body therapies showed that several mind and body exercise strategies are effective (2000). However, the number of randomized controlled trials in this review is limited. Yoga is one intervention that addresses both mental and physical characteristics. The practice of yoga can be roughly translated as the union of physical and mental or spiritual aspects of being. Yoga interventions consist of postures that promote awareness of the body in relation to the environment (i.e., proprioception), flexibility, balance, and breathing exercise. Yoga has been shown to reduce stress and promote relaxation (Telles, Reddy, & Nagendra, 2000; Vempati & Telles, 2002), improve sleep (Tooley, Armstrong, Norman, & Sali, 2000), retard coronary artery disease (Manchanda et al., 2000), and improve breathing, particularly in those with asthma (Manohcha et al., 2002).

Another study, a randomized controlled trial of patients with arthritis and carpal tunnel syndrome, showed that the practice of yoga improved functional performance, strength, and range of motion in addition to reducing pain (Garfinkel et al., 1998). Alleviating pain may facilitate the improvement of both physical and cognitive status (O'Connor, chapter 8) and ultimately prolong independence. Compared to wait-listed controls, those practicing yoga had better perceived energy, endurance, flexibility, sleep, and sex and social life and less loneliness as well as better mood and concentration (Blumenthal et al., 1989; Emery & Blumenthal, 1990).

In one of the few yoga studies that included older adults, volunteers with an average age of 72 who regularly participated in one of three types of activity were compared. One group ($n = 7$) engaged in proprioceptive physical activity, including yoga and soft gymnastics; another group ($n = 12$) practiced aerobic activity such as cycling, swimming, and jogging; a third group ($n = 21$) engaged in regular walking. The group practicing yoga and proprioceptive activities had the least sway on balance platform measures with eyes open and eyes closed. Although the aerobic group had the highest strength, they displayed poor postural control in comparison to the group practicing yoga. Both the aerobic and yoga groups had better balance than the walking group (Gauchard, Jeandel, Tessier, & Perrin, 1999). Although this study's design is weak, its results suggest that yoga may have benefits over and above usual activity (walking) or aerobic activity. Studies are needed in order to determine the multiple benefits of mind and body exercise on both physical and cognitive outcomes, and more research is needed on the safety and efficacy of yoga interventions in older adults.

Some Chinese exercises contribute to the overall well-being of an individual. Tai chi chuan, an ancient martial art form that originated in China thousands of years ago, continues to be practiced today. The goal of this discipline is to manage one's internal chi, which is the energy that is essential to the vital life force. Most of the randomized controlled trials that have utilized tai chi focus on balance and falls (O'Grady & Wolf, 2002). Qigong, another form of Chinese exercise that regulates chi, has many additional benefits. Management of gastrointestinal illness, arthritis, and ulcers are among the benefits from the few trials that have utilized this intervention (Luskin et al., 2000). Mind and body interventions, such as tai chi and qigong, have been found to improve balance, self-efficacy, and mental health as well as reduce the fear of falling (Kutner et al., 1997) and the incidence of falls (Province et al., 1995). Participants in tai chi chuan sustained a high level of interest and motivation to continue the program after the research project was over (Kutner et al., 1997). Mind and body exercise may have the added benefit of greater adherence than programs that address strength, endurance, flexibility, and balance separately. Failure to sustain levels of activity into late life is one of the reasons older adults have lower muscle mass and cardiovascular endurance (Marti et al., 1989).

Conclusion

Physical activity has beneficial effects on both physical and cognitive functioning in addition to alleviating psychological conditions such as depression and social isolation. Perhaps evidence of the ability of exercise training to alter disability is lacking because the interventions focus only on physical *or* cognitive effects but not both. In which case, studies are needed in order to determine the most efficacious exercise intervention for altering both physical and cognitive functioning. Perhaps mind and body interventions such as tai chi chuan or yoga can provide evidence of increased function in cognitive and physical arenas.

Mind and body exercise strategies may have a unique appeal for older adults for the following reasons: (1) Wise use of energy. Mind and body exercise has at its core a philosophy of energy cultivation through reducing stress and enhancing movement through better flexibility and range of motion. By comparison, endurance training is the intentional expenditure of calories, irrespective of skill development. Many, if not most, older adults want to conserve their personal energy in order to complete their daily activities. (2) Wise use of time. If mind and body exercise can address functional declines in both physical and cognitive function, the benefits per time expended stand to be greater when compared to engaging in activities that only contribute to one's individual strength, endurance, flexibility, balance, or other physical aspects. Time conservation is an important consideration for older adults who have difficulty accomplishing the necessary activities of daily living. (3) Desire to participate. Evidence suggests that mind and body interventions may engender a greater motivation to continue exercising.

Prolonged independence and high quality of life for the oldest old requires attention to internal capability in the context of overall demand. Three areas of research could provide guidance for developing strategies for late-life independence: (1) cognitive and physical markers of preclinical disability, (2) optimal intervention strategies to forestall dependency, and (3) tailoring individual environmental demand to match overall functional competency.

CHAPTER 8

Sleep, Mood, and Chronic Pain Problems

Patrick J. O'Connor, PhD

E xercise training has been proposed to influence cognition among older adults by acting on either primary or secondary aging (Spirduso, 1995). Primary aging is the aging that occurs in the absence of disease. To date, most experiments examining the influence of regular physical activity on cognitive functioning among older adults have involved individuals without disease (see chapter 7, Cress, on studies associated with diseases). The conclusion from this literature is that relatively short-term exercise training performed by older, healthy, sedentary individuals does not result in consistent or large improvements in cognition (see chapter 2, Tomporowski, and chapter 3, Poon and Harrington). Thus, the available evidence suggests that physical activity does not influence cognition among older adults by affecting primary aging.

This chapter makes a case that it is time for researchers to determine whether physical activity influences cognition via its effects on secondary aging. Secondary aging refers to diseases or environmental events that accelerate primary aging. There is evidence that reduced cognitive functioning among older adults is associated with health problems, including severe heart disease (Ahto et al., 1999), type 2 diabetes (Haan & Weldon, 1996), hypertension (Bohannon et al., 2002), sleep disorders, depression, and chronic pain.

Physical activity may influence elderly cognition through its effects on secondary aging. Three specific hypotheses are discussed in this chapter. The hypotheses are based on the supposition that exercise training can help attenuate age-associated cognitive impairment indirectly by improving components of health known to influence cognition. There is substantial evidence that exercise training is associated with improved health (Booth, Chakravarthy, Gordon, & Spangenburg, 2002; DiPietro, 2001); therefore,

I thank the following individuals for providing feedback about an earlier draft of this manuscript: Dane B. Cook, M. Elaine Cress, Phillip D. Tomporowski, and Shawn D. Youngstedt.

exercise training plausibly could indirectly help attenuate age-associated cognitive impairment by slowing secondary aging.

Hypothesis 1:
Exercise Training and Improvements in Sleep and Cognition

It is hypothesized that exercise training performed by older adults with sleep problems will attenuate age-associated cognitive declines by improving sleep.

Older Adults Sleep Poorly

A large number of cross-sectional studies have demonstrated that the prevalence of self-reported sleep problems increases with age (Bixler et al., 1979; Bliwise, King, Harris, & Haskell, 1992; Karacan et al., 1976). Compared to younger adults, older adults have changes in sleep architecture and a reduced total sleep time. The reduced total sleep time is caused by multiple factors including poor sleep habits, increased medication use, age-related changes in the circadian clock that contribute to early morning awakenings, and a higher prevalence of sleep disordered breathing (apnea) and periodic limb movements in sleep (Bliwise, 1993). Older adults have been found to be objectively sleepier during the day, and this is largely due to poorer sleep at night (Carskadon & Dement, 1992).

Poor Sleep Reduces Cognitive and Behavioral Functioning

As early as 1896, it was demonstrated that sleep deprivation impairs memory and reduces reaction time (Patrick & Gilbert, 1896). Over the subsequent century, large negative effects of acute (>30 continuous hours) and chronic (<5 hours of sleep per night) sleep deprivation on cognitive functioning have been observed (Dinges & Kribbs, 1991). In laboratory experiments, the most consistent effects of acute sleep loss have been short-term memory impairment and cognitive slowing (i.e., a reduction in the speed of responding to a wide variety of stimuli, but most especially during long-duration vigilance tasks).

Sleep problems appear to interfere with optimal cognitive performance by older adults. Several large studies of middle-aged (>50 years) and older (>65 years) adults (with sample sizes of 400 to 800) found that baseline subjective sleep complaints as measured by the Mini Mental State Examination predicted cognitive decline over a three-year period (Cricco, Simonsick, & Foley, 2001; Jelicic et al., 2002). Longitudinal research in which sleep was measured objectively in older adults who were at high risk for sleep disordered breathing ($n = 46$) found that increases in respiratory disturbances during sleep over a four-year period were significantly associated with decreases in cognitive performance as measured by the Mini Mental State Examination (Cohen-Zion et al., 2001). Moreover, sleep problems among older adults are thought to affect important "real world" cognition-dependent behavioral outcomes in a negative manner. For example, several investigations with large samples of elderly men and women (sample sizes ranged from 485 to 1,500) have found an independent association between reported sleep problems and falls (Brassington, King, & Bliwise, 2000; Schechtman et al., 1997).

Biological Basis Through Which Sleep May Influence Cognitive Processes

Sleep influences multiple brain areas involved in cognition. For instance, brain imaging studies using positron emission tomography have shown that during slow-wave sleep, neurons in the prefrontal cortex and the anterior cingulate cortex are less active than during periods of wakefulness. In contrast, during rapid eye movement (REM) sleep, there is increased neural activity in the hippocampal formation, anterior cingulate cortex, and in the posterior (temporo-occipital areas) cortices (Maquet, 2000). Other experiments have shown that brain areas activated during the day while completing cognitive tasks are reactivated during the subsequent night's REM sleep to a greater extent compared to control data (Louie & Wilson, 2001; Maquet et al., 2000). Investigations using electroencephalography with older insomniacs showed that reduced slow-wave sleep was associated with slower reaction times (Crenshaw & Edinger, 1999). These types of experiments have provided insight into the neurobiological bases for the role of sleep in human learning, memory, and psychomotor performance. Animal experiments also suggest that exercise training has effects on brain areas involved in cognition, sleep, mood, and pain (chapter 5, Holmes).

Exercise Training and Sleep Studies

Although there is not a large amount of literature on the effects of exercise on the sleep of older adults, several investigations show positive effects. Edinger and colleagues (1993) compared 12 physically active and aerobically fit older men to 12 sedentary older men. The fit subjects had shorter sleep onset latencies, less wake time after sleep onset, fewer sleep stage shifts during the initial portion of the night, less stage-one sleep, a higher sleep efficiency, and more total slow waves compared to the sedentary subjects. These differences in sleep architecture represent better sleep in the fit compared to sedentary subjects. Plausible alternative explanations for the results, such as better general health in the fit group, cannot be ruled out because of the cross-sectional research design used in this study.

Several longitudinal experiments have been conducted more recently. Singh, Clements, & Fiatarone (1997) conducted a randomized trial in which 32 depressed older adults (age 60-84 yrs) with poor sleep were randomly assigned to perform either weightlifting activities for 60 minutes, three days per week for 10 weeks or to engage in a health education control condition twice per week for 10 weeks. Overall sleep quality scores from the Pittsburgh Sleep Quality Index revealed that significantly more of the exercise program participants reported improved sleep quality after the intervention compared to those in the control condition.

Likewise, King and colleagues (1997) conducted a 16-week randomized trial in which 43 sedentary older adults (age 50-76 yrs) with sleep complaints either exercised (primarily walking) for 30 to 40 minutes, four times per week or maintained their usual level of inactivity. Sleep, as measured by both the Pittsburgh Sleep Quality Index and a sleep diary, was improved. Specifically, the time to fall asleep was reduced by an average of 15 minutes, and the total sleep time was increased by 42 minutes.

Additionally, a randomized trial compared one year of moderate-intensity walking exercise ($N = 45$) to nutrition education ($N = 40$) among sedentary older (age 62 ± 9 yrs) women family caregivers (King et al., 2002). Self-reported sleep quality was significantly better after one year of physical activity compared to the nutrition education condition. This is somewhat surprising given that sleep quality was not poor at the outset of the trial.

One investigation has examined the influence of increased physical activity on both objectively measured sleep and cognitive performance in a group of elderly people. Naylor and collaborators (2000) involved a group of 14 elderly (age 75 ± 3 yrs) residents of a continued-care retirement facility in a structured social intervention that included 20 minutes of light physical activity. The intervention was conducted from 9:00 a.m. to 10:30 a.m. and again from 7:00 p.m. to 8:30 p.m. daily for two weeks. A group of nine elderly residents served as controls. Following the intervention, the group involved in the structured activities had increased amounts of slow-wave sleep (~12 min) and demonstrated improvement in 10 memory-oriented tasks that was significantly better than the improvement shown by the controls. Although the greater improvement in cognitive function by the group that participated in structured activities was small in absolute magnitude (~4%), this investigation is notable because it underscores the potential relevance of the circadian timing of planned physical activity on health outcomes (Van Someren et al., 2002).

Conclusion

The research summarized in this section is consistent with the possibility that exercise training performed by older adults with sleep problems may attenuate age-associated cognitive declines by improving sleep.

Hypothesis 2:
Exercise Training and Improvements
in Depression and Cognition

It is hypothesized that exercise training by depressed older adults or those experiencing symptoms of depression will attenuate age-associated cognitive declines by improving symptoms of depression.

Many Older Adults Experience Symptoms of Depression

The six-month prevalence of a major depressive disorder, as defined by standard psychiatric criteria, occurs in about 0.4 percent of elderly men and 1.4 percent of elderly women (Myers et al., 1984). This compares to approximately 10 percent yearly prevalence among younger adults (Kessler et al., 1994). Symptoms of depression are much more common, with an average of approximately 15 percent of older adults scoring above symptom scale cutoffs suggestive of a clinical depression (Koenig & Blazer, 1992).

Depression Is Associated With Poor Cognitive Function Among Older Adults

It has been estimated that as many as 45 percent of persons age 85 years and older have significant cognitive impairment (Gallo & Lebowitz, 1999). Because the rate of depression among this age group is much less than 45 percent, it is obvious that depression is not the sole cause of reduced cognitive functioning with age. Nevertheless, cognitive impairment is common among depressed older adults as well as those reporting symptoms of depression.

A large number of studies have reported an association between increased symptoms of depression and reduced cognitive performance among older adults (Brown, Glass, & Park, 2002; Sato, Bryan, & Fried, 1999; Upadhyaya et al., 1999). Perhaps the strongest evidence of this type stems from longitudinal investigations in which higher symptoms of depression at baseline were found to be significant predictors of cognitive decline over several years (Cervilla, Prince, Joels, & Mann, 2000; Haynie et al., 2001). For example, Yaffe and colleagues (1999) prospectively followed 5,781 elderly, mostly white, community-dwelling women. Three cognitive tests (Trails B, digit symbol, and a modified Mini Mental State Examination) and the Geriatric Depression Scale were administered at baseline and four years later. Higher symptoms of depression at baseline were associated with worse performance at follow-up on all the tests of cognitive function. The authors concluded that depressive symptoms in older women are associated with both poor cognitive function and subsequent cognitive decline. If exercise training is associated with reductions in symptoms of depression, might this not also help attenuate age-associated declines in cognitive functioning?

Exercise Training and Depression Studies

Epidemiological investigations consistently have shown statistically significant, moderate, negative associations between self-reported physical activity and symptoms of depression among older adults (Camacho et al., 1991; Farmer et al., 1988; Mobily et al., 1996; Rajala, Uusimaki, Keinanen-Kiukaanniemi, & Kivela, 1994). Because this association might be explained by better general health among the more physically active individuals, it is essential to consider the results from randomized clinical trials concerning the effect of exercise training on depression.

Evidence from longitudinal experiments does demonstrate a link between increased physical activity and improvement in depressed mood among previously sedentary older adults. McNeil, LeBlanc, and Joyner (1991) studied 30 older adults (72.5 ± 6.9 yrs) who were mildly depressed. The participants were randomly assigned to a wait-list control, six weeks of walking twice per week with an undergraduate research assistant, or an equivalent time of social contact (talking, but not walking, with the research assistant). Scores on the Beck Depression Inventory (BDI) were reduced similarly in both the exercise and social-contact group but not in the wait-list control condition. The magnitude of the reduction in the somatic symptoms subscale of the BDI was about twice as large for the exercise group compared to the social-contact group. The findings suggest that exercise has larger effects on somatic symptoms of depression and that social interactions during exercise may contribute to improvements in depression symptoms.

Singh, Clements, and Singh (2001) randomly assigned 32 older adult (mean age of 71 yrs) outpatients with major or minor depression either to 10 weeks of supervised weightlifting exercise performed in a group setting followed by 10 weeks of unsupervised exercise or to 10 weeks of health education lectures followed by 10 weekly phone calls (control). The Beck Depression Inventory was administered before as well as 10 weeks, 20 weeks, and 26 months after the intervention. One-third of the exercise group continued to lift weights 26 months after the formal intervention had ended. Compared to the control group, the exercise group showed significantly decreased symptoms of depression after 20 weeks of exercise and at the 26-month follow-up. These findings are important because they show that the antidepressant effects of exercise can be realized with weightlifting, and these beneficial effects can be maintained for a long period of time among older adults who are willing to continue their exercise without supervision.

Blumenthal and colleagues (1999) randomly assigned 156 patients (mean age of 56) with major depressive disorder to 16 weeks of treatment using aerobic exercise, antidepressant medication (50-200 mg sertraline), or a combination of exercise and medication. The exercise program was performed in a group setting and involved 30 minutes of walking or jogging at 70 to 85 percent of heart rate reserve three times per week. Large decreases in psychiatrists' ratings of depression and in self-reported depression symptom scores were observed for all three conditions. These findings are important because they stem from a large randomized trial that compared exercise to a standard pharmacological treatment for depression. The results suggest that exercise is equally effective in reducing depression compared to a commonly prescribed selective serotonin reuptake inhibitor. Although this investigation of middle-aged adults did not show any advantages of combining exercise with medication, the results of a subsequent experiment did suggest that there may be advantages to combining the two treatments. Mather and colleagues (2002) studied 86 moderately depressed older adults (mean age of 68 yrs, 70% female) who had not responded to 6 weeks of antidepressant treatment. The patients were randomly assigned to either an exercise program or a health education program. Each program was conducted twice per week for 10 weeks. The exercise program entailed 45 minutes of weight-bearing exercise performed in a group setting while listening to music. The control condition involved attending health education talks that also were conducted in a group setting. All participants continued to take antidepressant medications during the experiment. After 10 weeks, a significantly greater percentage of the participants in the exercise group showed a large reduction in depression scores (a decrease greater than 30% of baseline) compared to the control group (55% vs. 33%).

Conclusion

The findings summarized in this section show that exercise training performed by depressed older adults is associated with improvements in depression. It is plausible that reducing symptoms of depression will contribute to improved cognitive function among older adults because depression and its symptoms are associated with poor cognitive functioning.

Hypothesis 3:
Exercise Training and Improvements
in Chronic Pain and Cognition

It is hypothesized that exercise training performed by older adults experiencing chronic pain will attenuate age-associated cognitive declines by reducing the frequency and intensity of the chronic pain.

Chronic Pain Is Common Among Older Adults

Many older adults suffer from chronic pain. Chronic pain can be defined as pain that persists for six months or longer. Chronic pain is often associated with marked negative behavioral and psychological changes including sleep disturbances and depression. The absolute prevalence rates of chronic pain vary dramatically among different studies (e.g., 10-80%), and this appears to be caused in part by the wide variations in the specific survey questions asked (Helme & Gibson, 1999). Nonetheless, epidemiological studies show that the overall prevalence of pain increases during adulthood from the second to the seventh decade. For example, in a telephone survey, Crook, Rideout, and Browne (1984) found that chronic pain was two to three times more prevalent among 60- to 80-year-old adults compared to younger adults in their 20s and 30s. The higher prevalence of pain is thought to be caused by the more frequent presence of physical pathology among older adults. Chronic pain among older adults is most commonly found in articular joints such as the knees, hip, and fingers, and this is associated with osteoarthritis (Andersson, Ejlertsson, Leden, & Rosenberg, 1993). Also, foot and leg pains increase markedly with aging. Obesity, diabetes, and peripheral vascular disease are primary contributors to chronic foot and leg pain among older adults (Benvenuti et al., 1995). The location of chronic pain is important with regard to exercise training interventions because the most common physical activity performed by older adults is walking. Pain in the foot, leg, knee, or hip can be a barrier to walking and other types of exercise performed by older adults.

Pain Reduces Cognitive Functioning

Older adults think that when they experience pain it interferes with their psychological functioning (Scudds & Ostbye, 2001). Moreover, empirical evidence obtained in several studies indicates that pain is associated with reduced cognitive performance. For example, in a study of 24 older adults (74 ± 7 yrs) who underwent spine surgery, a correlation of $r = 0.52$ was found between postsurgical pain and Trails A performance. This relationship was interpreted as indicating poorer cognitive processing speed among those reporting higher pain intensity (Heyer et al., 2000). Based on results from dozens of studies, reviewers have concluded that cognitive impairment occurs in patients with chronic pain, particularly on measures of attentional capacity, processing speed, and psychomotor speed (Hart, Martelli, & Zasler, 2000). Also, the weight of the available evidence suggests that the degree of cognitive impairment is related to the magnitude of pain intensity, with greater cognitive impairment more consistently occurring among people suffering from higher-intensity chronic pain.

Pain Is Represented in Multiple Brain Areas, Including Areas Involved in Cognition

Human brain imaging studies that involve exposure to noxious, painful stimuli have found increased neural activity in multiple brain areas. The most commonly activated areas include the thalamus, the somatosensory cortices S1 and S2, the insular cortex, and the anterior cingulate cortex (Casey, 1999; Derbyshire, 1999). The consistent involvement of the anterior cingulate cortex is important to the present discussion because the anterior cingulate cortex is thought to integrate affective, motivational, motor, and cognitive processes (Bush, Luu, & Posner, 2000; Paus, 2001). There is strong evidence that the anterior cingulate cortex is involved in attentional processes (Bush et al., 2000).

Chronic Pain May Influence Cognition Through Several Mechanisms

There are probably multiple mechanisms by which chronic pain alters cognition. One plausible mechanism is that pain competes for limited central nervous system attentional resources (Eccleston & Crombez, 1999). This idea accounts for the finding that the presence of high-intensity pain has larger negative effects on cognition if one accepts the notion that high-intensity pain requires more attentional resources than low-intensity pain (Eccleston, 1995). Also, a straightforward prediction from this hypothesis is that pain is more likely to affect a demanding cognitive task in a negative manner because of the greater attentional resources required.

There is clear evidence that depression impairs cognition in the elderly (King, Cox, Lyness, & Caine, 1995). Accordingly, a second plausible mechanism by which chronic pain reduces cognitive functioning is indirectly through its effects on depression. Perhaps the best data in this regard stem from a study in which multiple measures of pain, depression, and cognition were obtained from 121 community-dwelling arthritis patients age 34 to 84 (Brown, Glass & Park, 2002). It was found that individuals who performed poorly on the cognitive tasks were characterized by higher pain ($r = -0.27$) and higher depression scores ($r = -0.36$) and were older than those who performed well. Also, high levels of pain were significantly associated with depression scores ($r = 0.47$). Structural equation-modeling analyses showed that depression mediated the relationship between pain and cognition, even after controlling for age.

An overview of the negative influence of sleep problems on cognition among older adults was presented earlier in this chapter. This is relevant to a third possible mechanism by which chronic pain might negatively influence cognition; that is, by disrupting sleep. Numerous studies have reported that patients with chronic pain sleep poorly compared to those without chronic pain (Moldofsky, Lue, & Smythe, 1983; Smith et al., 2000; Wittig et al.,

1982). Perhaps the largest study of this type involved 429 men and women over age 65 with radiographic evidence of knee osteoarthritis (Wilcox et al, 2000). It was found that 31 percent of the participants reported problems falling asleep, 51 percent reported problems waking up too early, and 81 percent reported trouble staying asleep after falling asleep.

Exercise Training and Chronic Pain Studies

Relatively few experiments have been conducted examining the influence of exercise training on attenuating chronic pain among older adults. Koltyn (2002) has reviewed this literature and concluded that the strongest empirical support is for the effectiveness of exercise training in the management of osteoarthritis pain. Van Baar and colleagues (1999) have reviewed the randomized clinical trials concerning the influence of exercise training on osteoarthritis of the hip or knee. Most of the participants in these trials were older adults. Of 11 trials, 6 were found to be adequate in their research design. In these 6 trials, pain was reduced by a small to moderate amount. The authors argued that although firm conclusions could not yet be drawn because of the small number of well-designed experiments, there was evidence that exercise training had beneficial effects for patients with osteoarthritis.

Conclusion

The research summarized in this section is consistent with the possibility that exercise training performed by older adults with chronic pain problems may attenuate age-associated cognitive declines by reducing pain.

Conclusion

The American College of Sports Medicine's position concerning the consequences of physical activity for older adults concludes that the effects of exercise training on cognitive functioning are equivocal (Mazzeo et al., 1998). One plausible reason for the equivocal findings is that most investigators addressing the question have limited their recruitment of older research participants to those who are generally physically and mentally healthy. Although the decision to focus on healthy elderly is understandable, it may well have resulted in an underestimation of the potential effects of exercise training on attenuating age-related declines in cognition. The weight of the available evidence suggests that physical activity does not influence cognition among older adults by affecting primary aging. Physical activity may influence cognition by reducing secondary aging (Spirduso, 1995); however, this idea has been inadequately tested to date.

The information presented in this chapter argues that it is time for investigators to conduct randomized trials of the effects of exercise on cognition in which older adults with health problems known to affect their cognitive functioning in a negative manner are recruited. This approach has been employed with those suffering from chronic obstructive pulmonary disease (Emery, 1994; Emery, Leatherman, Burker, & MacIntyre, 1991; Emery, Schein, Hauck, & MacIntyre, 1988; Etnier & Berry, 2001). However, cognitive impairments have been reported to be small among this patient group (Fix et al., 1982). Nonetheless, this type of approach will allow us to learn whether physical activity can be an effective tool in combating age-related declines in cognition by alleviating major health problems, such as poor sleep, depression, and chronic pain, afflicting older adults.

CHAPTER 9

Brain Blood Flow and Methodological Considerations

Kevin McCully, PhD, and Yagesh Bhambhani, PhD

B rain metabolism is rather unique in that it is dependent on the oxidative metabolism of glucose. Aging is associated with altered or reduced cognition, with inadequate delivery of oxygen or glucose being implicated in these conditions (Donohoe & Benton, 2000). The high metabolic rate of brain tissue and the essential nature of oxidative metabolism are associated with a complex arterial system serving the brain. About 75 percent of the blood going to the brain comes from the two common carotid arteries. The common carotids divide into internal (servicing the brain) and external (servicing facial muscles) branches. The remaining blood to the brain comes from the two vertebral arteries. There are a number of interarterial connections in the head that can minimize the negative effects of a major block in one of the arteries. In contrast to arteries going to skeletal muscles, the arterial circulation of the brain is a low-resistance system in which the arteries are continuously dilated, and in which there is little sympathetic tone or flow modulation (Kremkau, 1998). Despite this, cerebral blood flow is highly regulated. The purpose of this review is to evaluate the approaches used to measure blood flow to the aging human brain. The review will consist of a brief overview of age-related changes in blood flow, followed by a presentation of techniques that have been used to measure blood flow to the brain. In particular, two methods, Doppler ultrasound and near-infrared spectroscopy (NIRS), will be presented in detail.

Age-Related Changes in Blood Flow in Healthy Individuals

There are a number of ways that aging could influence blood flow to the brain. Most of the evidence for age-related changes in blood flow has been obtained from peripheral vessels. Structural changes in blood vessels, such as altered arterial diameters or stiffer vascular walls, could occur (figure 9.1). Both of these have been reported to occur within older subjects

(Bortolotto et al., 1999). Venous compliance and response to central volume change was reported to be altered in older compared to younger subjects (Olsen & Lanne, 1998). Reduced venous compliance will reduce the ability of older humans to respond to changes in central blood volume. Control of blood flow could also be altered because aging has been associated with increased sympathetic tone (Ziegler, Lake, & Kopin, 1976). Similarly, augmented forearm vasoconstriction during dynamic leg exercise has been reported in healthy older men, although response to cold pressure test was blunted (Taylor, Hand, Johnson, & Seals, 1992). This could result in lower-than-required blood flow during activities that alter blood flow such as standing up (postural challenge) or exercise. Reduced flow and vascular conductance were reported during cycle ergometry exercise in younger and older subjects carefully matched for fitness levels (Proctor et al., 1998). There is some evidence that control of distribution of blood flow can be altered with age. Redistribution of blood flow as measured by skin blood flow was reduced in the elderly during exercise (Kenney & Ho, 1995). Aging is associated with reduced vascular health, as defined by reduced communication between vascular endothelium and vascular smooth muscle (Smith, 2001). However, total blood flow capacity to skeletal muscle may not be decreased with age (Olive, DeVan, & McCully, 2002), so it is unclear how functionally significant the reported age-related changes are. It should be noted that aging can also reduce the oxygen-carrying capacity of the blood or alter glucose regulation so that metabolism can be impaired even with normal blood flow.

Blood Flow With Age:
Cardiovascular Disease

Cardiovascular disease is an age-associated disease, increasing in prevalence with age. The primary mechanism behind cardiovascular disease is occlusive atherosclerosis, although it can also result from arterial aneurysms and inflammatory vasculitis (Mann, 1983). Mortality from cardiovascular disease occurs primarily from atherosclerosis in blood vessels in the heart and brain. Occlusive atherosclerosis seems to occur primarily at arterial branch points and may be facilitated by alterations in shear stress at these points (Smith, 2001). Atherosclerosis is a progressive disease, but symptom severity can progress in a nonlinear fashion (Humphries, deWolfe, Young, & LeFevre, 1963). A major impact of cardiovascular disease on research in the elderly is that the almost universal prevalence of some degree of atherosclerosis makes it difficult to dissociate "healthy" age-related changes in circulation for those associated with disease.

A number of risk factors influence the prevalence and severity of atherosclerosis. These include smoking, presence of diabetes, physical inactivity,

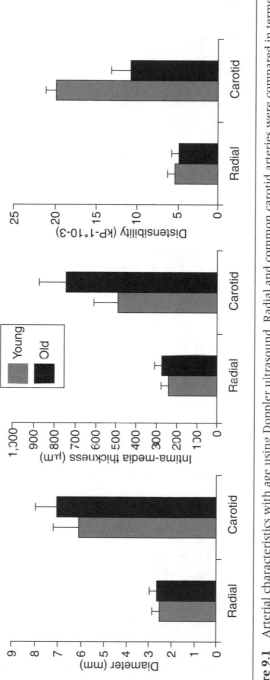

Figure 9.1 Arterial characteristics with age using Doppler ultrasound. Radial and common carotid arteries were compared in terms of vessel diameter (left), vessel wall thickness (center), and vessel distensibility (right). Age resulted in significant alterations in the carotid but not the radial arteries.

Reprinted, by permission, from L. Bortolotto et al., 1999, "The aging process modifies the distensibility of elastic but not muscular arteries," *Hypertension* 34: 889-892.

hypertension, hypercholesterolemia, and family history of vascular disease. Increased central fat was associated with increased sympathetic nervous system activity in young and old men (Poehlman et al., 1995). Acute intake of high-fat meals may impair vascular function (Vogel, Corretti, & Plotnik, 1997), although not all studies support this finding (Djousse et al., 1999). African Americans have higher rates of cardiovascular disease than Caucasians. Age-adjusted mortality from stroke was found to be 76 percent higher in African American men and 54 percent higher in African American women than in Caucasian counterparts (Dwyer, 1995). Endothelial function also seems to be reduced in older African Americans compared to Caucasians (Ergul, Tackett, & Puett, 1999). African Americans have reduced endothelial nitric oxide release (Cardillo, Kilcoyne, Cannon, & Panza, 1999). However, race is a complex factor, with contributions from differences in genetics and the environment (Baker, 1999; Clark, 1995).

Sex is also an issue in the prevalence of cardiovascular disease because men have a higher initial incidence of disease, which evens out as people get older. In a group of subjects who were either at risk for type 2 diabetes or had uncomplicated type 2 diabetes, the women had greater vascular reactivity than the men (Caballero et al., 1999). Women may have reduced ability to vasodilate (Martin et al., 1990), and different capacities of vascular control (nitric oxide pathways) than men (Ergul, Shoemaker, Puett, & Tackett, 1998). Thus, blood flow measurement of the brains of older subjects may be very population dependent.

Methods Used
to Assess Brain Blood Flow

Measurement methods can be divided into those that evaluate blood flowing through large vessels (blood flow) and those that measure flow through small vessels (typically termed perfusion). Studies of healthy humans need to be noninvasive, although a number of minimally invasive methods have been used. Minimally invasive can refer to administration of tracers (usually but not always radioactive) through cannulation of veins or inhalation and signal detection using high-energy sources such as X rays. [133]Xenon is an example of a free diffusible tracer that is used with single photon emission computed tomography (SPECT) and contrast computed tomography (CT) to evaluate brain perfusion (Owler & Pickard, 2001). Both approaches provide localized brain perfusion measurements, although assumptions need to be made concerning the partition of the tracer in various tissues in the brain, and quantification of the measurements is difficult. Positron emission tomography (PET) uses tracers such as $H_2{}^{15}O$ and ${}^{15}O$ to measure brain perfusion and oxygen extraction. Thus, PET provides information on blood flow and tissue metabolism. All of the tomography measurements are limited by relatively long data collection periods, so they are not practical for dynamic measurements.

Magnetic resonance imaging (MRI) has developed into a powerful and versatile tool to evaluate brain blood flow and perfusion (Bihan, 1994; Roberts, Kehayias, Lipsitz, & Evans, 1993). MRI uses the relationship between magnetic fields and radio frequencies to measure radio frequency signals emitted from protons, usually in water molecules. From these signals, detailed anatomical information, blood flow in large arteries, tissue perfusion, water diffusion coefficients, and oxygen content can be measured. Although MRI blood flow measurements are enhanced with the use of contrast agents, anatomical and perfusion measurements can often be done without them. No administration of a contrast agent and the use of low-energy radiofrequency make MRI noninvasive.

Functional MRI (fMRI) is a technique to monitor activity-related changes in regional oxygen content (Ellermann et al., 1994). This is a popular approach that can measure dynamic changes in brain function. Areas of the brain that have increased activity also have increases in blood oxygen levels that affect proton relaxation rates and can be detected with fMRI. The advantages of MRI are that it can have the best available spatial resolution (for anatomical measurements) and can monitor changes in brain activity. The disadvantage of MRI is that it requires the use of large expensive magnets and spectrometers, and especially with fMRI, it requires expert technical help to perform the experiments.

Doppler Ultrasound Measurements of Arterial Blood Flow

Doppler ultrasound uses sound waves that can image the diameter of an artery and can measure blood velocity (Kremkau, 1998). Brightness mode (B-mode) images use the amount of sound that bounces off interfaces between tissues of different densities, such as the blood vessel wall and blood itself, to obtain an image of the blood vessel. Spectral imaging records the magnitude in the shift in sound frequency as sound travels through a blood vessel to determine blood velocity. If both measurements are made at the same time (duplex imaging), blood flow can be calculated. Doppler ultrasound can be performed on the middle cerebral artery in the head (referred to as transcranial Doppler) and on the major arteries in the neck (common carotid, internal and external carotids, and vertebral arteries). The advantages of Doppler ultrasound are that, in addition to being noninvasive, Doppler ultrasound can provide continuous information about blood flow as well as the size and wall thickness of the arteries. The disadvantage of Doppler ultrasound is that it is sensitive to movement, which makes measurements during exercise difficult (but not impossible).

A number of studies have used Doppler ultrasound to assess blood flow to the brain in older humans. The middle cerebral artery is considered to be the best available marker of cerebral blood flow with Doppler ultrasound. However, the middle cerebral artery is technically difficult to study (Nagai, Kemper, Earley, & Metter, 1998). Nagai and colleagues (1998) used transcranial Doppler in 498 older subjects and were able to obtain adequate signals from 75 percent of them. The transcranial Doppler technique uses a small easy-to-place probe that can perform spectral but not B-mode imaging. Thus transcranial Doppler does not provide information on vessel diameter and can only be used to measure blood velocity. Success rates for Doppler of the middle cerebral artery that included diameter measurements were even lower (Nagai et al., 1998). To obtain a higher success rate for blood flow measurements (approximately 97%), the common carotid has been used as an index of brain blood flow (Nagai et al., 1998). The disadvantage of using the common carotid artery is that it includes blood flow to the external carotid, which mostly services noncerebral tissue in the head.

As shown in figure 9.2, the internal carotid and external carotid arteries respond very differently to facial muscle exercise and postural challenge. This is similar to what has been seen in response to rapid pressure changes in the common carotid compared to the temporal superficial artery (Savin, Siegelova, Fisher, & Bonnin, 1997). In addition, approximately 25 percent of total brain blood flow is provided by the vertebral arteries (Scheel, Ruge, Petruch, & Schoning, 2000; Seidel, Eicke, Tettenborn, & Kurummenauer, 1999). In some subjects, the vertebral arteries are smaller than normal (termed vertebral hypoplasia). It is also possible that compensation could occur in the vertebral arteries in subjects with reduced carotid blood flow (Seidel et al., 1999). This suggests that investigations of brain blood flow might need to include measurements of all the major arteries, rather than just using one as an index of total flow. A key issue in the use of Doppler ultrasound is the difficulty of the method. Experienced technicians are needed and careful attention to experimental details is required for consistent and reliable results. The conclusion from these studies is that the common carotid artery might be a practical way of assessing cerebral blood flow, but that using a more specific artery, such as the internal carotid, might be better.

Doppler ultrasound studies have reported age-related declines in carotid and middle cerebral artery blood velocity. Scheel, Ruge, and Schoning (2000) reported a decline of approximately 0.4 percent per year starting in a person's 20s. In some studies this decline was not seen in the vertebral arteries. In addition, the ratio of artery thickness to internal diameter decreased, indicating increasing wall thickness. Increasing wall thickness is consistent with findings of greater arterial stiffness with aging. This was evident in subjects without known carotid artery pathology, although Perret and Sloop (2000) found that hypertension in the range of 130 to 160 mmHg was associated with increased blood velocity. This result suggests

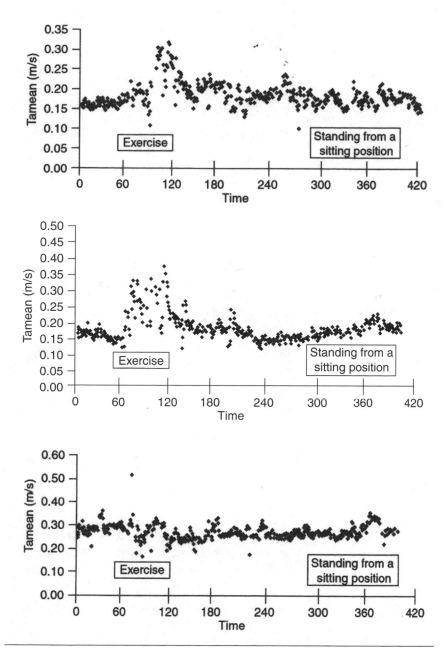

Figure 9.2 Representative examples of arterial blood flow during exercise and postural challenge. Top: left common carotid artery. Middle: left external carotid artery. Bottom: left internal carotid artery. Exercise consisted of jaw clenching. Postural challenge consisted of moving from sitting to standing position. Note that internal carotid artery services the brain and shows smaller responses to exercise and postural challenge than the external carotid that services facial muscles. Time is in seconds.

that blood pressure can be an important determinate of brain blood flow, at least in certain ranges. Doppler ultrasound has not been used to monitor brain blood flow during exercise because of the difficulty of overcoming movement artifacts.

Near-Infrared Spectroscopy Measurements of Brain Oxygen Saturation

Another rapidly developing technique for evaluating brain oxygen saturation is NIRS (Chance et al., 1989; McCully & Hamaoka, 2000). NIRS is based on the differential absorption properties of chromophores (light-absorbing compounds) in the near infrared region between 700 nm and 1,000 nm (Simonson & Piantidosi, 1996). The known chromophores that absorb infrared light in the tissues are hemoglobin (Hb), myoglobin (Mb, only in muscle), and cytochrome oxidase. In muscle tissue, significant signals come from Hb and Mb. Signals from hemoglobin and myoglobin cannot currently be differentiated because the absorbency spectra of these two chromophores overlap in the near infrared range.

For studies of brain tissue, the lack of Mb simplifies the interpretation of the NIRS signals to just that of Hb. At 760 nm, Hb and Mb occur mainly in the deoxygenated form (deoxyHb and deoxyMb respectively), whereas at 850 nm, they occur in the oxygenated state (oxyHb and oxyMb respectively). The difference in tissue absorbency between these two wavelengths indicates the relative change in Hb/Mb oxygen saturation in the tissue capillaries. The sum of the absorbencies at these two wavelengths indicates the relative change in localized blood volume that is independent of changes in hematocrit. One of the limitations of NIRS is that absolute muscle oxygen uptake cannot be accurately quantified because the absolute path length of the NIRS signal cannot be determined (Simonson & Piantidosi, 1996). Therefore, changes in oxygenation and blood volume relative to the resting baseline value are usually used for analysis. However, current studies report absolute results on skeletal muscle from carefully selected subjects (usually with little body fat) for which the same correction factors are generally applicable (Quaresima, Colier, Sluijs, & Ferrari, 2001; van Beekvelt et al., 2001).

Validity and Reliability of Cerebral Near-Infrared Spectroscopy

The use of NIRS in the brain has been primarily to place the NIRS device on the frontal lobe of the cerebral cortex. This is due to the practical considerations of gaining access to upper brain centers while avoiding hair. This limits the use of NIRS to monitoring expected changes in the frontal cortex (in people who have hair on their heads). It has been difficult to assess the utility of NIRS in monitoring brain oxygen levels because of the difficulty of using other methods to measure oxygen saturation of small vessels in the brains of intact humans (Simonson & Piantidosi, 1996). Nonetheless, a number of studies have been used to validate the use of NIRS in tracking skeletal muscle oxygen saturations and blood volumes. For the brain, highly significant correlations between the changes in jugular bulb venous oxygen saturation (an index of mixed cerebral oxygenation) and NIRS determined changes in cerebral oxygenation. Such correlations have been reported in healthy subjects inspiring oxygen concentrations ranging from 6 percent to 13 percent under resting conditions (Pollard et al., 1996).

Other evidence has indicated a significant relationship between total hemoglobin change measured by NIRS and cerebral blood flow at different penetration depths determined by PET during cerebral activation (Villringer et al., 1997). Comparable results have also been demonstrated in the cerebral cortex during rhythmic handgrip exercise that is measured simultaneously by magnetic resonance spectroscopy and NIRS (Kleinschmidt et al., 1996). Similar trends have been reported in cerebral blood volume measured by transcranial Doppler and cerebral hemodynamics measured by NIRS in healthy subjects and patients with spinal cord injury (Houtman et al., 2001).

However, not all studies have supported the validity of NIRS. Buchner, Meixensberger, Dings, and Roosen (2000) concluded that NIRS measurements were not useful in studying cerebral oxygen levels after acute brain injury. This was primarily due to the high rate of test failure and a limited sensitivity.

Cerebral Oxygenation and Blood Volume Trends Measured by NIRS

During the last few years, researchers have applied NIRS to examine acute changes in cerebral metabolism under a variety of conditions such as visual, cognitive, and motor stimulation (Obrig & Villringer, 1997). Depending on the type of stimulus, the NIRS probe is placed on the occipital lobe (visual), temporal-frontal lobe (cognitive), or frontal lobe (motor). During motor stimulation tasks, the NIRS probe is usually placed on the right or left frontal lobe, approximately 3 cm from the midline and 1 cm above the supraorbital ridge (figure 9.3) (Kleinschmidt et al., 1996; Obrig et al., 1996). The underlying assumption for cerebral NIRS is that the increase in neuronal activation during functional tasks is linked to an overall increase in cerebral oxygenation and blood volume (Dirnagl, 1997). The phenomenon of neural activity increasing oxygen saturation is also what is detected with fMRI.

Postural challenge results in greater decreases in oxygen saturation in the cerebral cortex of older subjects than in younger subjects (figure 9.4)

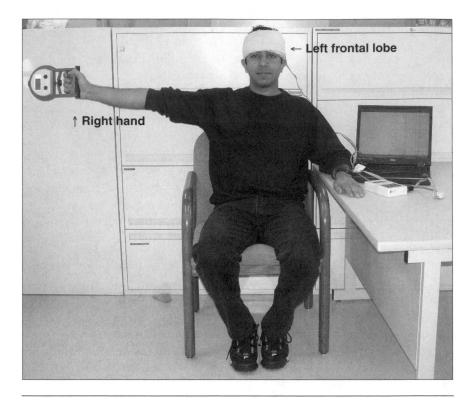

Figure 9.3 Setup for NIRS measurements of cerebral oxygenation and muscle oxygenation during exercise. The probe is carefully placed over the left frontal cortex and covered to minimize contributions from extraneous light sources. In this example, isometric exercise is performed with the right arm using a handgrip dynamometer.

(Mehagnoul-Schipper et al., 2000). In older men ranging from 70 to 84 years, the orthostatic changes on two separate occasions demonstrated poor reliability coefficients of the oxygenated and deoxygenated forms of hemoglobin, although the direction of the responses was similar on both occasions, and no significant interaction between test and time was found (Mehangoul-Schipper, Colier, & Jansen, 2001).

In another study that evaluated the NIRS responses during head-up tilt in healthy males, a small reproducibility error was reported for stroke volume, mean arterial pressure, and deoxygenated hemoglobin (Houtman, Colier, Hopman, & Oeseburg, 1999). However, there was a higher error for oxygenated hemoglobin and total blood volume measured by NIRS. Older subjects with documented postural hypotension (abnormally reduced blood pressure with standing) had greater changes in oxygen saturation with standing than nonaffected subjects (Harms et al., 2000). In poststroke

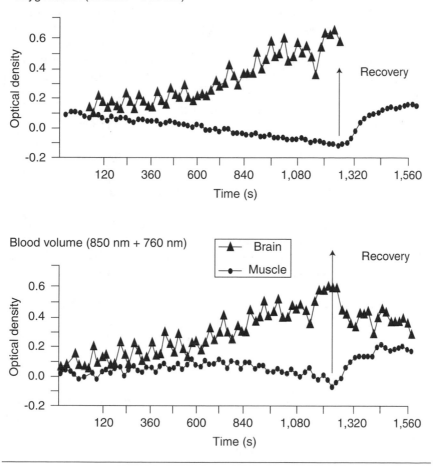

Figure 9.4 Brain oxygenation changes with postural challenge.

Reprinted, by permission, from J. Mehagnoul-Schipper et al., 2000, "Cerebral oxygenation declines in healthy elderly subjects in response to assuming the upright position," *Stroke* 31: 1615-1620.

patients, changes in brain oxygen saturation were associated with different cognitive and motor tasks including head-up tilt, mental calculations, listening to music, and walking (Saitou et al., 2000). The different tasks seemed to be associated with unique changes in blood volume and oxygen saturation.

Physical Activity and Cerebral Oxygenation and Blood Volume Measured by NIRS

Several studies have used NIRS to evaluate cerebral oxygenation and blood volume trends during a variety of motor stimulation tasks. Obrig and colleagues (1996) evaluated the NIRS trends in 56 healthy subjects performing a finger movement task for 10 seconds. They observed significant increases in blood volume and oxygen saturation over the left frontal lobe during this task. The increase in oxygen saturation was accompanied by a corresponding decrease in deoxyhemoglobin concentration. Further, the cerebral NIRS response increased with the frequency of the motor stimulus, and the magnitude was greater when the task was performed on the contralateral side compared to the ipsilateral side. Colier, Quaresima, Oeseburg, and Ferrari (1999) studied the cerebral NIRS response during easy and difficult hand and foot movements (in-phase and antiphase respectively) and demonstrated significant increases in cerebral oxygenation and blood volume during these tasks. However, they were not able to demonstrate significant differences in these trends associated with task difficulty.

Recently, several investigations have demonstrated that NIRS can be used to evaluate changes in blood volume and oxygen saturation during hypoxia and dynamic exercise such as rowing, cycling, and treadmill walking and running. Saito and colleagues (1999) demonstrated that cerebral NIRS measurements taken from the forehead were sensitive to changes in arterial hypoxia induced by altitude exposure. In 10 healthy office workers with no mountain trekking experience, they demonstrated a significant decrease in cerebral oxygen saturation (calculated as the ratio between blood volume and oxygen saturation) during three minutes of stepping exercise at altitudes of 2,700 m and 3,700 m compared to sea level. The decline in cerebral oxygen saturation was proportional to the decrease in arterial oxygen saturation at the different levels of altitude. Ide, Horn, and Secher (1998) demonstrated that blood volume and oxygen saturation increased systematically during cycling exercise, with the changes being proportional to the exercise intensity—between 30 percent and 60 percent of the maximal oxygen uptake. These observations were consistent with the blood flow observations determined simultaneously from the middle cerebral artery using transcranial Doppler.

Several studies have used NIRS to simultaneously examine regional changes in cerebral and muscle hemodynamics during exercise. The oxygenation and blood volume trends during stepwise incremental cycle exercise to voluntary fatigue in a representative healthy male subject are illustrated in figure 9.5. It is evident that the trends in both of the NIRS variables are different in brain and skeletal muscle. In cerebral tissue, blood volume and oxygen saturation increase linearly with exercise intensity and in a parallel manner until $\dot{V}O_2$max is attained. During recovery from exercise, the cerebral response is variable. Some subjects demonstrate a rapid decline toward baseline values, whereas in others, both cerebral oxygenation and blood volume tend to remain elevated for several minutes after the cessation of exercise. In the vastus lateralis muscle, oxygenation

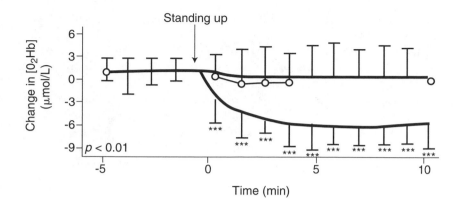

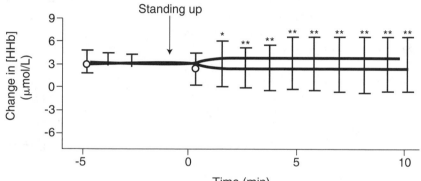

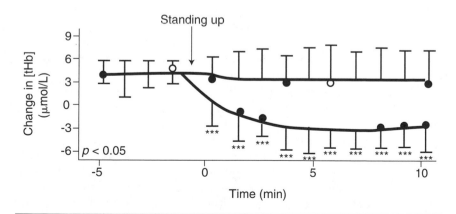

Figure 9.5 Cerebral oxygenation and cerebral blood volume trends measured by near-infrared spectroscopy in a representative subject during stepwise incremental cycle exercise to voluntary fatigue.

progressively decreases during stepwise incremental exercise with a leveling off as the $\dot{V}O_2$max is attained.

Some researchers (Belardinelli, Barstow, & Wasserman, 1995; Grassi et al., 1999) have demonstrated an exaggerated decline in skeletal muscle oxygenation at the lactate or ventilatory threshold. The increased rate of desaturation has been attributed to the accumulation of lactate in the blood that tends to shift the oxyhemoglobin curve to the right via the Bohr effect (Wasserman, Hansen, & Sue, 1991). This facilitates the release of oxygen from the oxyhemoglobin complex so that it can be utilized in the mitochondria for energy production. During incremental exercise, muscle blood volume increases to approximately 50 to 60 percent of the maximal oxygen uptake; then it tends to level off until voluntary fatigue is attained. During recovery from dynamic exercise, muscle oxygenation recovers very rapidly during the first minute and usually demonstrates a large hyperemia. This increase tends to level off during the recovery period, with the values returning to near baseline levels after several minutes of recovery. Muscle blood volume returns to resting levels during the recovery period but takes several minutes to reach the preexercise level.

Nielsen, Boushel, Madsen, and Secher (1999) used NIRS to examine simultaneously the regional changes in muscle and cerebral oxygenation in elite rowers during a six-minute maximal rowing effort. The results indicated that vastus lateralis muscle oxygenation decreased significantly during maximal rowing, as expected. Cerebral oxygen saturation from the left frontal lobe indicated a decline from 82 percent at rest to 65 percent during maximal exercise. The researchers attributed this to a significant decrease in the arterial oxygen saturation from 98 percent at rest to 91.9 percent during maximal exercise. When these experiments were repeated under hyperoxia (inspired oxygen concentration of 30%), oxygen saturation was maintained during maximal exercise, and the decline in cerebral oxygen saturation observed under normoxic conditions did not occur.

In another study, Nielsen, Boesen, and Secher (2001) used spatially resolved NIRS to simultaneously study regional changes in the deoxyHb and oxyHb concentration of the vastus lateralis, biceps brachii, intercostals, and frontal lobe during submaximal and maximal cycling with resistive breathing. The results indicated that breathing against resistance induced a significant increase in the ventilation rate, while oxygen saturation and end-tidal carbon dioxide tension were significantly reduced. These trends were reversed when the breathing resistance was removed. Whole-body oxygen consumption at all levels of resistive breathing was not significantly different from the control (unresisted breathing) condition. Low to moderate resistive breathing did not alter the vastus lateralis and intercostal deoxyHb concentration compared to the control condition. However, intense resistive breathing induced a significant increase in vastus lateralis and intercostal deoxyHb concentration. Cerebral deoxyHb and oxyHb concentrations increased significantly as a result of moderate and intense resistive breathing, along with elevated blood volume. The authors suggested that carbon dioxide production during exercise regulates regional blood flow to both the active muscles and the brain, with a more modest effect on the muscle tissue.

Conclusion

Brain blood flow is an important factor in determining brain function. Aging, either "healthy aging" or in association with cardiovascular disease, can have a significant impact on brain blood flow. A number of different methods of measuring brain blood flow have been used in various studies. In particular, Doppler ultrasound has become popular because of its modest cost, noninvasive nature, and its ability to provide continuous information on blood velocity and vessel diameter. NIRS, a developing technique for measuring brain blood flow, has the advantage of being relatively inexpensive, portable, and noninvasive. A number of studies have shown NIRS to be a sensitive technique for evaluating changes in tissue oxygenation and blood volume during functional tasks and whole-body exercise. In particular, older subjects have been shown to have reduced control of blood oxygen saturation with postural challenge. However, quantification of NIRS signals awaits further technical developments, and several NIRS studies have reported difficulties with measuring cerebral oxygen saturation. Doppler ultrasound has become the method of choice in monitoring blood flow in and to the brain, despite the difficulty in using it during exercise. NIRS has been used successfully to monitor changes in frontal cortex oxygen saturation with postural challenge and motor and cognitive tasks. However, several studies have produced inconsistent findings, perhaps related to the difficulties in quantifying NIRS signals. Thus, NIRS is a promising method that needs further development.

CHAPTER 10

Neuroimaging in an Aging Population: Potential Tools in Cognition, Everyday Functioning, and Exercise Research

L. Stephen Miller, PhD

The main goals of this chapter are to describe several modern neuro-imaging techniques, particularly functional neuroimaging, and review their use in aging research. The chapter also very briefly describes neuro-imaging in exercise research and discusses the potential for neuroimaging techniques as tools to study the relationship between cognition, functional ability, and exercise in older adults.

The last three decades have seen an explosion in technologies for directly viewing the anatomy and function of biological systems, including neural systems thought to regulate human behavior. Prior to the 1970s, there were only very limited methods of viewing the structure of the brain and central nervous system (CNS), primarily through the use of simple X rays. Although X rays have been an invaluable source of information regarding the morphology of anatomical structures, particularly bone, they have not been particularly effective in differentiating soft-tissue differences inherent in brain structure. Interestingly, there has been a longer history of measurement of *functional* brain activity, primarily through the use of electroencephalography (EEG), which dates back to Hans Berger in the 1920s (Berger, 1969). EEG has successfully allowed for real-time measurement of brain activity and, while not a primary focus of this chapter, is discussed briefly in later sections.

I want to thank Drs. Keith Becker, Gene Binet, Joseph Borelli, and Lawrence Tannenbaum, and GE Medical Systems for their generous permission to reproduce several of the figures in this chapter.

Nevertheless, it is only recently that significant advances in visualization of the brain and its function have occurred. Techniques including computerized tomography (CT) and magnetic resonance imaging (MRI) have resulted in the exquisite *in vivo* visualization of brain structures (as well as other body tissue) in incredible detail. Advances in these structural technologies have also resulted in the development of exciting new methods of visualizing real-time or near real-time brain function, including positron emission tomography (PET) and the related single photon emission computerized tomography (SPECT) as well as functional magnetic resonance imaging (fMRI). Finally, following on the success of EEG, the technology of magnetoencephalography (MEG), a measure of the magnetic fields created by the electrical activity of the brain, has recently been used to measure brain function. Together, these techniques offer opportunities to increase our understanding of both the specific morphology of the brain and its functional underpinnings.

The next few pages present briefly several major neuroimaging techniques, including in basic terms how they work; how they present data regarding anatomy, morphology, and function; their current typical uses; and some of their limitations. Following this is a synopsis of how neuroimaging has been used to increase our understanding of aging within the nervous system.

Neuroimaging of Brain Structures

The visualization of the human brain through noninvasive neuroimaging techniques has revolutionized our understanding of this most complex of all human organs; some of these techniques are summarized below. For an extensive review of neuroimaging techniques, the reader is directed to *Brain Mapping* by Mazziotta, Toga, and Frackowiak (2000).

X Ray

X-ray imaging (radiography) has been an available research tool for some time. First discovered by Wilhelm Roentgen before the turn of the 20th century (Nitzke, 1971), X rays are energy beams of very short wavelengths (0.1-1,000 Å) that are made up of high-energy photons (particles of light). Thus, they are a form of electromagnetic radiation, just like visible light. X rays are able to penetrate most substances, and the amount of penetration is dependent on the density of the substance exposed. Specially designed machines can pass X rays through organic material, including living organisms. When X rays are passed through the body, differences in contrast are developed via a photographic process so that images reflecting different material density are produced. High-density materials such as bone allow few photons to pass through and appear bright white. Places that con-

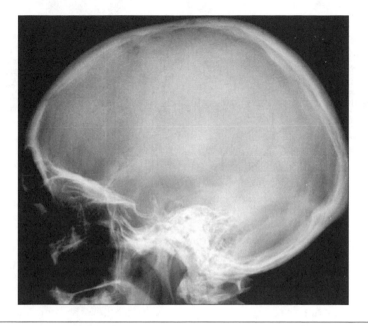

Figure 10.1 Typical skull X ray of a healthy older adult male.

Courtesy of Dr. Gene Binet.

tain little tissue or a great deal of air appear black. Materials of moderate density (e.g., soft tissue like muscle or fat or liquids) appear as variable shades of gray. The ability to use this high-penetrance electromagnetic radiation technique provides a wealth of information about bone trauma, tissue abnormalities, and observance of certain kinds of tumors and other disease states. Sometimes, high-density agents (contrast agents) are used in conjunction with X-ray technology to enhance the contrast between certain structures (e.g., arteries) and surrounding tissue. Contrast agents are selected to block photon penetration and thus appear bright white on film. Figure 10.1 illustrates the X-ray film with which most of us are familiar.

In the area of aging, X-ray technology allows for the study and recognition of age-related changes such as decreased bone density, organ shrinkage, and, when using contrast agents, arterial or venous system obstructions and occlusions, among others. In the study of pathological changes, X rays are similarly helpful in recognizing acute changes. In older adults, X rays have been used in the study of bone fractures, osteoporosis, arterial blockage, tumor identification, lung damage, pneumonia, heart disease, hydrocephalus, sinusitis, seizures, meningitis, and even certain types of dementia.

However, the resolution of the X ray is not as high as that of newer techniques, including CT and MRI. This lack of resolution has been particularly limiting for X-ray use as a measure of brain anatomy. Brain (and nervous) tissue, although varying somewhat in density, generally is too uniform for a standard X ray to denote significant differences in subtypes of tissue. Additionally, standard radiography is a two-dimensional technique. Still, it is an inexpensive, painless, relatively noninvasive, and easily performed technique that presents a detailed picture of many body materials and identifies many common problems.

Although beneficial, X rays are not without their risks. When photons pass through the body, most are absorbed in the cellular tissue and the energy can negatively affect that tissue. Although most of the damage at the cellular level is not permanent, some loss of cellular integrity occurs. Thus, X-ray exposure is regulated, and radiation exposure should be limited.

CAT: Computerized Axial Tomography

Computed tomography (CT) or computerized axial tomography (CAT) techniques are essentially very specialized radiography procedures. Using X rays, they represent a computer-based assembly of multiple X-ray images. However, rather than being a single exposure taken through large areas of tissue, CT scanning represents a series of thin cross-sectional (planar) images or slices taken at, or nearly at, the same time. Rather than the X-ray system sending a large burst of photons through the body as in conventional X rays, the CT system is composed of one or more pairs of X-ray sources and "detectors," which result in multiple thin planar slices of tissue being evaluated. These thin slices are a great improvement over conventional X rays because of the vast reduction in the amount of tissues that are superimposed one on another. This in turn greatly reduces the scatter effect found in conventional X rays.

Data are collected as the system moves around the person being scanned, with scans being taken at many different angles through tissue areas. The X-ray source or detector pairs produce multiple images from these different angles, which are then reconstructed by computer programs and made available as two- and three-dimensional image sets. As a result of these multiple angles and images, averaging techniques can be used, resolution is vastly improved over conventional X rays, and contrasts have a much finer grain (see figure 10.2). This results in higher spatial resolution as well.

CT does a much better job than conventional X rays in identifying different types of tissue and can be used to image most major soft tissues including internal organs, muscle, fat, and nervous tissue. It has become relatively inexpensive, is quick and efficient, and is readily available in most medical settings. CT imaging of the head and of the brain is used to detect and differentiate tumors. Blood clots are readily seen, and blood vessels can be imaged quite well, enabling the identification of defects within vessels. The anatomy of the brain can be imaged with significant clarity, and differences between gray and

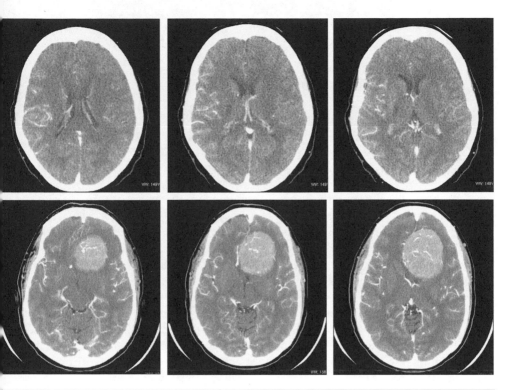

Figure 10.2 CT scan examples. Top: Midaxial brain view of a 45-year-old male showing right "luxury" perfusion, a hyperperfusion most likely resulting from an embolic stroke. Bottom: Midaxial brain views of a 63-year-old male showing a large left frontal meningioma. Radiological convention with left and right sides reversed.

Courtesy of MRI at Belfair.

white matter and between brain and nonbrain tissue can be seen. Contrast agents, which are inert substances that increase the contrast between normal and abnormal tissues, are sometimes used in CT imaging.

Using CT images to identify pathology in the brain has greatly increased our understanding of the function of the brain because we can correlate behavioral performance to specific brain structures or brain damage. Because CT images are computer collected, the postprocessing capabilities are great. This enables reconstruction of images from multiple angles and three-dimensional image reconstruction. These images can then be used not only for detection but also for intervention strategies such as guidance in surgical procedures.

As would be expected in the study of aging, CT has been used to identify age-related changes with excellent results. It has been used to image soft tissue, as X rays have, but with greater contrasts and spatial resolution. CT has also been used to assess brain pathology in older adults. Tumors, brain atrophy or degeneration, and cerebrospinal fluid are all important targets of CT scanning. Perhaps one of the most important uses has been its ability to detect blood hemorrhages. CT has a nearly 100 percent detection rate for brain hemorrhaging, a common sequelae of stroke.

As in X-ray technology, there are some risks to CT. These include exposure to radiographic photons, which cause problems similar to conventional X-ray exposure. However, total exposure is less for CT.

MRI: Magnetic Resonance Imaging

Along with CT, magnetic resonance imaging (MRI) makes up the majority of brain imaging technologies in use today (Mitchell & Cohen, 2004). MRI is a noninvasive imaging technique that uses magnetic fields and radio-frequency energy to affect atomic nuclei. Thus, it is quite different from CT imaging. MRI was first developed from nuclear magnetic resonance (NMR) research in the mid-1970s (Lauterbur, 1973). Like CT, the object is to produce a series of cross-sectional planar images that show contrast differences across tissue types. Unlike CT scanning, X rays are not used. Instead, MRI passes a strong magnetic field through the tissue of interest in order to detect spin phenomena of subatomic particles. Hydrogen is most often targeted because it is abundant in biologic tissue and its nucleus is a single proton. This results in a strong signal.

Protons naturally spin and thus produce individual magnetic fields. However, in normal circumstances they are randomly oriented in their natural biological environment, and thus, the overall magnetic field of any given tissue area is neutral. When exposed to a strong magnetic field, these protons align (orient) with the external magnetic field. However, alignment is not perfect and each spinning proton rotates "around" the direction of the applied magnetic field. This movement around is most often described as being similar to a top as it spins and is called the "precess."

Using a radiofrequency (RF) field applied to the tissue, the orientation of the protons with the magnetic field can be temporarily moved (the "flip angle"). Once this RF field is removed, the protons return to their normal orientation within the external magnetic field ("relaxing"). In doing this, they release the RF energy they had absorbed under the RF field. This released RF energy and subsequent relaxation of the proton from the resultant flip angle can be detected by an RF receiver as a signal change. Differences in the temporal gradient (duration) of this relaxation suggest different proportions of the hydrogen protons and thus differing tissue. Images are therefore based on these proportional differences in overall signal changes as a result of spin relaxation.

All tissues of the body have specific proportions of hydrogen atoms; therefore, their images are somewhat unique. For example, on a standard

T1-weighted image, greater proportions of hydrogen in tissue show up darker than tissues with less hydrogen. Thus, water-saturated tissues, such as those seen in edema or hemorrhaging, produce a low signal and show up very dark, while water-reduced tissues such as fat produce a high signal and show up very bright. Intermediate tissues such as brain tissue show up in varying contrasts, again dependent on hydrogen proportions. MRI has no equal in terms of spatial resolution, routinely producing images at the submillimeter level. As magnet strength continues to increase and postprocessing computer programs continue to improve, so too will the spatial resolution of MRI.

As in CT scanning, collections of planar images are combined by computer programs to "reconstruct" the tissue of interest in two- and three-dimensional space. The final result of MRI technologies is a very fine, detailed picture of anatomy as can be seen in figure 10.3, a 3 tesla–based high-field sagittal image of the human brain. It can be used to assess the structure of most biological tissue and is useful in most cases where tissue anatomy is in question. MRI has been used to look at nearly every human organ and tissue type: cardiac tissue, muscle tissue, lung tissue, and brain and spinal cord tissue. It is especially helpful in imaging tissue of the central nervous system (CNS), brain, and spinal cord. Because of its high resolution, it is often the neuroimaging technique of choice when looking for tumors or other pathological structures in the CNS (see figure 10.4).

Additionally, certain pathological processes involved in neurological disorders are best seen by MRI. These include subtle atrophy or degeneration of brain volume, smaller metastatic tumors, certain kinds of intracranial vascular lesions, protein disturbances (e.g., plaques) specific to multiple sclerosis, and features of Parkinson's disease. In clinical and research studies of aging, MRI has been particularly useful in studying and

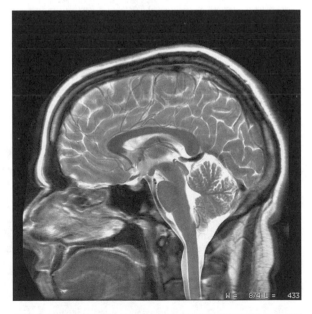

Figure 10.3 High-field sagittal-view T1 MRI scan of the human brain, illustrating the exquisite detail possible.
Courtesy of GE Medical Systems.

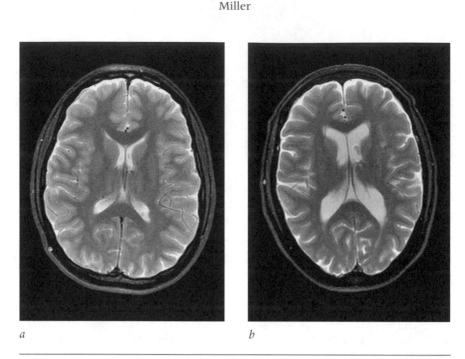

a   b

Figure 10.4 High-field (3T) MRI axial view scans. *(a)* Normal 32-year-old female with complaints of headache. *(b)* 62-year-old male with complaints of memory difficulties (note atrophic sulcal areas and enlarged ventricles).

Courtesy of MRI at Belfair.

describing these neurological abnormalities because they are some of the most common health changes that occur in older adults. MRI additionally has the advantage of not using ionizing radiation.

Another great advantage of MRI is its flexibility. MRI technologies have been developed that allow the imaging of certain chemicals in the CNS. This specialized form of magnetic resonance imaging (magnetic resonance spectroscopy [MRS]) uses the MRI technology to assess the anatomical dispersion of certain chemicals, often neurotransmitter substances or their precursors or metabolites. As such, MRI has the potential to explain the chemical changes occurring in the brain during cognitive activity. MRI can also be adapted to gather detailed images of the entire blood system (magnetic resonance angiography [MRA]). Finally, MRI measures can be adapted to obtain indirect measures of functional brain activity (fMRI).

All available evidence suggests that the magnetic field exposure in MRI is generally harmless to body tissue. However, the process has some risks. First, the magnetic field can accelerate ferrous-based objects toward the center of the magnet. Thus, ferromagnetic objects must be kept out of the MRI room and away from the magnet. This includes ferromagnetic materials within soft tissue such as metal fragments in the eye. Because signal differences are produced by rapidly changing the magnetic field, under certain circumstances voltage currents can be generated as a consequence in materials that are electroconductive and whose conductor is in a closed circuit. As a result, closed circuits such as those found in a pacemaker should be excluded from the MRI environment. Finally, RF pulses can generate localized heat within body tissue if unregulated, causing tissue damage in extreme cases.

Neuroimaging of Brain Function

While structural imaging (as discussed in the previous sections) has extricated much of the mystery surrounding the neuroanatomical aspects of the human brain, it tells us little about *how* the brain performs its marvelous functions. Functional neuroimaging techniques are beginning to allow us a glimpse into the mechanisms of these processes. Following are descriptions of several of the most prominent functional neuroimaging techniques.

PET: Positron Emission Tomography

Positron emission tomography, or PET, is a technique that measures the absorption or accumulation of trace amounts of radioactive-labeled chemicals that have been placed into the bloodstream. Their distribution and subsequent absorption into tissue is measured and converted into two- and three-dimensional images reflecting that distribution. Specifically, certain naturally occurring chemicals, most often glucose or oxygen or sometimes analogs of those compounds, can be "labeled" or "tagged" with a radioactive component. This "radiotracer" is then injected into the bloodstream and becomes distributed to areas of the body in which that compound is normally distributed or metabolized. Sensors of the PET scanner are able to detect the radioactivity as the compound is distributed to different tissues. PET measures the decay properties of the chemical used as a release of positively charged particles called positrons.

These data are used to reconstruct the distribution of the compound by computer software, resulting in images of that distribution. In the case of glucose, sensors detect the radioactive-labeled glucose as it moves from the injection site through the arterial system of the brain. Areas that accumulate larger amounts of labeled glucose are presumably using more glucose, a measure of brain activity (figure 10.5). Recently, radiotracers have been developed that can be embedded into additional brain chemicals such as certain neurotransmitters. In this way, it is possible to map out the specific binding sites of these neurotransmitters *in vivo*.

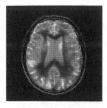

Figure 10.5 PET-FDG scan of a 70-year-old male with mild Alzheimer's disease, superimposed on his axial MR T1-weighted image. Note hypometabolism in anterior temporal and posterior parietal regions.

Courtesy of Johnson and Becker.

The advent of PET neuroimaging has opened up a whole new set of methodologies for understanding the functions of the brain in real time. Because it measures chemical processes such as blood flow or glucose metabolism, PET allows inspection of changes in the chemical processes of the brain resulting from both normal and abnormal functioning. Hence, one can look at normal metabolic processes during cognitive activities (e.g., remembering a string of words) in order to assess which areas of the brain are using energy during those activities. Also, one can look for changes that occur while engaged in a cognitive task following a brain change, such as disease or insult. Prior to PET, cognitive function had been inferred from behavioral changes, which were often apparent only after considerable disease progression. With the advent of PET, detection of chemical changes such as glucose utilization provides much earlier information in the time course of a disease. Spatial resolution of PET is moderate, with perfusion study resolution down to the order of 5 mm^3.

PET has been used extensively in the study of aging. In brain insult (e.g., trauma, tumors, epileptic foci), hypometabolism is frequently seen. In degenerative and dementing illnesses, hypometabolism has been seen in a variety of cortical and subcortical regions (e.g., Mazziotta, 1989; Mazziotta, Frackowiak, & Phelps, 1992). Research regarding normal aging changes has primarily been researched by simple comparisons of the cognitive abilities of younger and older people. Findings have generally supported a generalized hypometabolic process of brain activity in older versus younger adults. It is presumed that this hypometabolism reflects synaptic loss, deficits in energy metabolism, or a reduction in glucose transport.

The use of fast-decaying radioactive tracers in PET has advantages and disadvantages. The advantages are that they allow for fairly rapid measurement; thus, brain function that occurs in this short time frame can be measured. For example, radioactive-labeled oxygen has a half-life of about two minutes. The disadvantage of this is the need for expensive and highly specialized equipment to prepare these tracers, such as a cyclotron, designed to accelerate and then capture hydrogen ions for radioisotope production. Additionally, PET neuroimaging is not without some risks. These include exposure to small amounts of radioactivity, as well as small risks of infection caused by involvement of a foreign substance in the blood stream.

SPECT: Single Photon Emission Computed Tomography

Single photon emission computed tomography, or SPECT, is similar to PET in that it uses radioactive tracers with a similar detection system to reconstruct images of activity occurring in the brain. SPECT has actually been in use longer than PET. However, images are less detailed, and rapid changes in brain function cannot be observed because of the tracers used. Nonetheless, SPECT has a long history of being used to study the neurotransmitter dopamine.

Unlike PET, which measures positron emission, SPECT uses specialized detectors, or gamma cameras, to record photon emission from radioactive tracers injected into the blood supply to the brain. Thus, it can be a measure of cerebral blood perfusion, or regional cerebral blood flow (rCBF). However, SPECT also takes advantage of special tracers that are absorbed into the brain tissue itself via the blood supply system. SPECT uses radioactive tracers that have a longer shelf life than typical PET tracers, and several are commercially available. These tracers are ones that freely cross the blood–brain barrier (BBB) and remain fixed within the brain without significant redistribution long enough for SPECT images to be collected. Most of these tracers (e.g., Iodine 123-IMP) quickly move across the BBB and remain distributed for 20 to 60 minutes. Simply put, the radioactive tracer over time gathers in brain regions in relation to the rate of blood flow to that brain region. Detectors measure photon emission in these areas in real time to give a measure of the amount of rCBF. This is then inferred as representative of functional activity of those brain regions that have taken up the tracer. A specialized type of SPECT scanning sometimes used is an inhalation method of the radioactive tracer [133]Xenon to measure rCBF. Unlike other tracers, [133]Xenon clears the brain very rapidly, allowing multiple studies to be performed.

Because SPECT images are collected over many angles, they can be computer reconstructed in any two-dimensional or three-dimensional space. This allows for SPECT images to be "coregistered" with CT or MRI scans. Coregistered images then give information about structural morphology and functional activity in the brain.

Advantages of SPECT include the reduced expense and expertise needed for conducting the studies compared to PET or fMRI, as is discussed later. Also, longer-lasting radioactive tracers are used, making them better products for storage without specialized manufacturing procedures; on the other hand, PET usually needs a cyclotron in the facility to prepare the shorter-lived radioactive compounds.

Limitations of SPECT include a somewhat lower level of resolution than PET, although the newer multidetector systems used in research settings have spatial resolution approaching the quality of PET systems (approximately 10 mm full width). Additionally, SPECT has a reduced ability to image deeper brain structures because photons are attenuated as they pass through tissue.

SPECT has been used for some time in the study of aging, similar to PET. It has proven especially useful in the measurement of dopamine distribution, important in a variety of age-related disorders such as Parkinson's disease. It has also been successfully used in identifying ischemic insult.

fMRI: Functional Magnetic Resonance Imaging

Functional magnetic resonance imaging, or fMRI, uses many of the same principles of standard MRI. However, rather than focusing on the magnetization properties of hydrogen, fMRI uses measurement of the magnetic properties of oxygen during times of brain activity. Images are based on the indirect measurement of activity in the brain through comparisons of magnetization changes caused by blood flow, blood volume, and oxygen saturation. This is known as the blood oxygen–level dependent (BOLD) method (Ogawa, Lee, Nayak, & Glynn, 1990; Ogawa et al. 1993).

The typical BOLD fMRI strategy is to compare the amount of oxygenated hemoglobin in the microvascular system in specific brain regions during a particular brain activity to those same oxygen levels during inactivity. When a brain area is "activated," blood flow increases to that site. This results in a proportional change of oxygenated blood within the microvasculature, particularly the venous system, of that area. This occurs within a few seconds, tapering off after several more seconds. This magnetic susceptibility change can be compared to the magnetic susceptibility of the local blood oxygenation when the brain area of interest is "at rest" through subtraction methods. In comparison, periods of less activity have relatively greater deoxygenated levels of blood, which has different measurable magnetic properties.

fMRI has a multitude of advantages over other functional imaging techniques. Compared to PET and SPECT, the spatial resolution is much greater, with accurate resolution near 1 mm^3. Thus, the image clarity is far superior. Because the data is collected using MRI techniques and equipment, concomitant MRI structural images can be collected, giving very precise coregistering capabilities. Together, fMRI and MRI provide exquisitely sensitive images of functional activity of the brain and precise placement of that activity on the morphological MRI images.

fMRI is currently being used in aging research primarily to assess changes in cognitive activity following brain insult from degenerative states such as Alzheimer's disease. It is also being used in direct comparisons of younger versus older persons' cognitive performance (see figures 10.6 and 10.7). Data suggest that older adults may have altered or adapted activation of brain regions while engaging in cognitive tasks compared to younger persons.

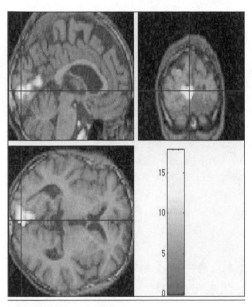

Figure 10.6 fMRI example of older adult brain activation presented with right visual field stimulation.

Reprinted from Miller et al., 2002.

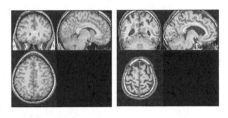

Figure 10.7 Coronal, sagittal, and axial views of young (left) and older (right) adult brain activation differences during a stimulus interference task (Stroop task). Also note the structural differences, including sulcal and ventricular size.

Reprinted from Miller et al., 2003.

fMRI, like MRI, is seen as a safe, noninvasive method of *in vivo* research into the workings of the brain. However, the same risks of MRI are inherent in fMRI exposure.

Electromagnetophysiological Techniques (EEG, ERP, MEG)

These technologies—electroencephalography (EEG), event-related potentials (ERP), and magnetoencephalography (MEG)—are all based on summative information of very large aggregates of neurons. They have the advantage of high temporal resolution, approximately a few ms, but relatively poor spatial resolution. EEG and ERP measure electrical activity associated with neuronal firing characteristics, while MEG measures the very small magnetic field changes occurring during neuronal activity. Because of the high temporal resolution, these techniques allow research questions concerning the relative timing of events and can give important information regarding connectivity and direction of neuronal activity. They have been somewhat limited by the poor depth of signal detection because electrodes are usually based on measures from the scalp. In some settings, for example surgical interventions, electrodes can be temporarily placed in deeper brain structures for increased spatial resolution.

EEG allows spontaneous neuronal activity measurement (Prinz, Dustman, & Emmerson, 1990), while ERP allows system-based study by measuring the electrical potentials elicited by presented stimuli (e.g., motor, sensory, or cognitive information). They are thought to reflect dendritic activity within upper-cortical cell layers (Glaser, 1963). MEG provides similar temporal resolution with somewhat greater spatial resolution. EEG and ERP data have primarily been used to quantify neuronal processing changes by defining architectural changes in the major frequency bands: alpha, beta, theta, and delta. It has also been used to assess changes in functional independence of cortical areas in older compared to younger adults (Dustman, Emmerson, & Shearer, 1996). A discussion of these functional techniques is beyond the scope of this chapter; interested readers are directed to the comprehensive review by Dustman and colleagues (Dustman, Shearer, & Emmerson, 1993).

Neuroimaging As a Tool for Aging Research

Chapters 1 through 3 have specifically addressed the relationship between cognition and aging, and these relationships will not be outlined in detail in this chapter. Suffice it to say that there are a host of age-related changes that cognitive testing has shown. These include, for example, decreases in crystallized intelligence (Schaie, 1989), recall memory (Smith, 1996), speed of information processing (Hertzog & Bleckley, 2001), and inhibitory control (Sweeney, Rosano, Berman, & Luna, 2001). However, until recently, structural and functional origins of these age-related changes had been difficult to quantify. The advent of neuroimaging techniques has allowed researchers to study the relationships between these cognitive changes and specific changes in the brain. Both structural and functional neuroimaging techniques have helped in these studies. Recently, explanatory models regarding these changes have used structural and functional neuroimaging as components (e.g., Cabeza, 2001, 2002; Cabeza, Anderson, Locantore, & McIntosh, 2002).

Examples of Structural Neuroimaging Tools in Aging

There are many structural neuroimaging contributions to our understanding of cognitive changes in aging. Both pathological aging processes and natural age-related processes have been investigated. Beginning with CT brain scanning introduced in the 1970s and followed by MRI in the 1980s, relationships between brain morphology and cognition have been studied. It is now clear that predictable volume decreases in brain tissue are a result of the natural aging process (Blatter et al., 1995). This relationship is exacerbated not only by pathological processes of aging such as the degenerative dementias but also by other injuries such as head and brain trauma and vascular compromise.

Thanks to neuroimaging techniques, we have begun to identify more specific information regarding this tissue loss and have been able to characterize the type of loss and, to a certain extent, its regional specificity. Structural neuroimaging techniques have shown that volumetric changes are primarily due to corresponding ventricular enlargement and reductions in the gray matter (Pfefferbaum et al., 1994; Raz et al, 1997) and have further substantiated the decrease in brain volume with decreases in a host of cognitive abilities. Information regarding specific brain regions has also been gathered and, though less consistent, has given us information helpful in understanding their relationship to cognitive change. For example, the hippocampus and the broader structures of the hippocampal formation are considered important areas for memory function. Hippocampal structural changes in healthy aging have been seen by some researchers (e.g., Jernigan et al., 2001; Small et al., 2000) and are related to memory performance (Golomb et al., 1994).

These findings have not been universal, however, and at least one study has suggested that hippocampal volume remains relatively stable (Good et al., 2001). Recent research has suggested that white matter undergoes relatively minor changes over time (Miller, Alston, & Corsellis, 1980; Sullivan et al., 2002). Furthermore, Jernigan and colleagues (2001) have suggested that white-matter tissue stays relatively stable for much of the aging process, then quickly declines after age 70. When white matter changes are seen, they have been seen in some but not all brain regions (Guttmann et al., 1998; Jernigan et al., 2001). Good and colleagues (2001) reported anterior frontal white matter and the posterior limbs of the internal capsule, a major fasciculus in the brain, showing greater age-related volume loss compared to posterior frontal areas, cerebellum, and temporal lobes. From these studies, we have been able to develop a picture of the aging brain that, although variable from person to person, indicates a slow tissue loss over time. This tissue loss is greater in areas of cell body accumulation (gray matter) and generally does not affect white matter tracts until later ages. When white-matter loss is seen, it is likely seen in anterior brain regions to a greater extent than posterior regions.

Because of its prevalence in older adults, progressive dementing illnesses such as Alzheimer's disease (AD) have been the focus of a great deal of aging research. Because treatment of Alzheimer's and related progressive dementias appears to produce a better outcome if begun early in the disease process, much effort has gone into the early detection of disease. Cognitive measures alone, although important in identifying AD, are far from perfect in their ability to distinguish AD from normal aging changes (Chen et al., 2000). Structural neuroimaging techniques have been used to assess the morphological changes of the brain as a result of these pathologies.

Both CT and MRI have been important in documenting these changes. For example, CT combined with histological data has demonstrated temporal lobe atrophy in the middle stages of AD (Brun & Englund, 1981). However, high-resolution MRI is the current state-of-the-art technology. Studies have shown that persons suffering from Alzheimer's disease clearly show hippocampal formation and overall medial temporal lobe tissue loss. This loss appears to correlate with the degree of memorial impairment seen in these individuals. Of much interest currently is the use of high-resolution MRI to differentiate mild or early Alzheimer's disease from normal aging changes. Again, the hippocampal formation has been targeted by many researchers.

Two relatively new techniques, voxel-based morphology (VBM) (Ashburner & Friston, 2000) and cortical mapping (e.g., Mazziotta et al., 2001), allow for the automatic quantification of high spatial–resolution MRI scans by analyzing physiological variability across an entire coordinate system or specific coordinates of three-dimensional MRI maps of the brain. Using VBM and cortical mapping techniques, researchers have discriminated persons diagnosed with mild Alzheimer's disease from healthy age-matched controls based on hippocampal morphological differences (Csernansky et al., 2000; Haller et al., 1996; Rombouts et al., 2000). These appear primarily as volume differences but, because of their precision, have the benefit of being able to separate relatively small hippocampal structures from one another. A group of researchers in particular, Small and colleagues (2000), have used specialized, very high spatial–resolution MRI techniques to compare resting-state activity (function) in the hippocampal formation substructures of early AD patients and healthy age-matched controls. Their findings indicate that different substructures differed in the amount of activity compared to controls. Significant differences between controls and early AD patients were found in entorhinal cortex, subiculum, CA1, and the dentate gyrus-CA3 grouping, with the greatest difference found in the resting-state activity of the entorhinal cortex.

The studies discussed earlier and many more like them offer support of structural neuroimaging as effective in measuring both natural and pathological age-related changes in brain morphology. Furthermore, these studies indicate a relationship between these brain changes and cognitive performance deficits. Although causal data largely remain lacking, the current body of structural neuroimaging literature indicates a significant association between these two variables. In fact, Mega, Thompson, Toga, and Cummings (2000), in their review of brain-mapping techniques in dementia, state that the combination of brain-mapping techniques, cognitive performance, and risk factors is the best predictor of Alzheimer's disease in older adults with mild cognitive impairment (MCI).

Examples of Functional Neuroimaging Tools in Aging

Other than the electrophysiological methods, PET, SPECT, and fMRI have been the primary techniques in studying functional changes in real-time brain processes. Each has advanced our understanding of functional abilities in aging as they relate specifically to brain activity, and the data is presented here somewhat interchangeably between the functional imaging techniques. First, however, it is important to review the fundamental differences between structural and functional neuroimaging techniques.

Unlike structural neuroimaging techniques, which measure morphology *in isolation* of task performance, functional techniques such as PET and fMRI measure *brain function* as a reflection of behavioral task performance. This means that there are significant conceptual differences between the kinds of questions asked between structural imaging and functional imaging methods. As summarized by Fletcher (2000), structural techniques allow the comparison of cognitive deficits (e.g., through neuropsychological testing) and independent measures of brain morphology. Although this is limiting in terms of the inferences that can be made, it is fairly straightforward, as seen in some of the earlier examples, and has given strong support to a relationship between cognitive performance deficit and a host of brain pathologies.

On the other hand, functional neuroimaging techniques utilize the experimental approach of manipulating an independent variable (e.g., age) and observing changes within some dependent variable (e.g., functional activity) in a particular brain region. As such, the components and properties of the experimental tasks have an impact on the dependent measure (e.g., function) and our interpretation of those tasks. Functional neuroimaging can only inform us about brain and behavior relationships to the extent that the behaviors (i.e., tasks engaged) are consistent with the measures of brain activity that we use (e.g., glucose utilization in PET, BOLD changes in fMRI). These assumptions are far from being unequivocally supported by the literature. These are pointed out not to negate functional neuroimaging as a valuable tool, but to serve as a gentle caution in comparing findings from structural imaging to those findings in functional imaging and in remaining cognizant of problems that can influence the interpretation of functional neuroimaging results.

As outlined in the previous section, structural neuroimaging, particularly high-resolution MRI, has been invaluable in our detection of both developmental aging changes and pathological changes such as Alzheimer's disease. As noted earlier, however, discrimination between the two has remained somewhat limited because of the considerable similarity between natural age-related brain morphology changes and the early pathological changes of the AD process. Hence, study of functional changes holds promise in giving us value-added information.

This chapter first presents functional imaging research as it pertains to our understanding of normal age changes in cognition and follows this with examples of functional imaging studies that have focused on pathological aging effects on cognition.

Normal Studies

The earliest functional neuroimaging studies of normal aging used PET resting-state functional imaging techniques (e.g., deLeon et al., 1984; Frackowiak, Lenzi, Jones, & Heather, 1980). Metabolic PET studies have not been entirely consistent (e.g., Itoh et al., 1990), but have generally found small but statistically significant reductions in cortical metabolism in a variety of regional brain areas from aging. These reductions have ranged from about 1 to 8 percent per decade (Blesa et al., 1997). Perfusion PET studies have shown similar but more variable results of decreased rCBF (Martin, Friston, Colebatch, & Frackowiak, 1991; Pantano et al., 1984). Thus, resting-state studies indicate that in normal aging there is likely an overall linear decline in metabolic and cerebral blood flow to the brain related to increased age. This has been most often interpreted as reflecting the general biological changes underlying cognitive differences between older and younger adults. However, virtually all of this work is correlational in nature.

Functional activation studies of normal aging have been much more recent, with the first studies in the early 1990s using PET to assess differences in visual perception among young and old groups (e.g., Grady et al., 1994; Madden et al., 1997). PET has remained the primary functional neuroimaging technique to study normal aging changes. These PET studies generally demonstrated that older adults showed weaker activation on visual face and location tasks in primary visual areas but greater activation than younger adults in anterior activity, particularly prefrontal cortex. Secondly, activity within the anterior regions was more bilateral in older than younger adults (Grady et al., 2000). This observation has been interpreted as a dysfunction in the ventral and dorsal pathways of the visual system, with older adults being less able to recruit early visual system information, resulting in an increased reliance on higher-order brain regions. This is consistent with well-established findings of improved elder performance at the cost of performance speed. Work in our laboratory (Miller, Bedwell, Allison, & Strauss, 2002) indicates that on simple tasks of visual perception, where visual stimuli are presented to one visual field at a time, older adults show slightly less overall intensity and fewer overall numbers of activated voxels in the expected contralateral visual cortex, but show greater bilateral activation in other regions (see figure 10.7).

In complex cognitive tasks such as memory encoding, older adults have shown varying differences in activation of hemisphere-specific processing depending on the task, when compared to younger adults. In tasks of semantic-based encoding, less activity has been found in the left prefrontal cortex (PFC) and left temporal lobe compared to younger adults in general combined with greater right hemispheric activity in a variety of regions including right PFC and the right insula (Grady et al., 1995; Madden et al., 1996). Similarly, tasks of word encoding, which contain a significant attentional component, show less left PFC activation but greater right PFC activation in older adults (Anderson, Iidaka, et al., 2000; Cabeza et al., 1997).

Conversely, in a number of studies of episodic retrieval, less relative activation has been typically found in right PFC and other right hemisphere regions combined with greater left PFC in older compared to younger adults (Anderson et al., 2000; Cabeza et al., 1997; Madden et al., 1999). Similar findings are seen in working memory tasks, with hemisphere-specific tasks showing relatively less PFC activation and commensurate increased bilateral activation (e.g., Grady et al., 1998; Reuter-Lorenz et al., 2000) and in tasks of inhibition (e.g., Miller, Bedwell, Yanasak, & Allison, 2003). Together, these findings are consistent with a model of age-related decreases in lateralized function (Tulving et al., 1994).

Cabeza has recently summarized these findings (Cabeza, 2001, 2002) and offered an explanatory model. Cabeza presents the overall reduction of PFC lateralization as the hemispheric asymmetry reduction in old adults (HAROLD) model. This model, in simple terms, states that as we age, we rely less on hemisphere-specific control of cognition and rely on greater bilateral control. This finding is consistent with a long-held view of greater resource use as a compensatory mechanism for age-related cognitive changes (e.g., Craik & Byrd, 1982). Cabeza and colleagues (2002) have taken the HAROLD model one step further in attempting to test two divergent hypotheses of how this decreased lateralization comes about. Decreased lateralization as we age may be related to either (1) compensatory mechanisms or (2) deficit in neuronal recruitment of specialized neurons. Cabeza and colleagues (2002) have termed these as the compensatory hypothesis and the dedifferentiation hypothesis, respectively. Although data exist to support the dedifferentiation hypothesis (e.g., Baltes & Lindenberger, 1997; Li & Lindenberger, 1999; Mitrushina & Satz, 1991), recent neuroimaging data appear to support better the compensatory hypothesis (Cabeza et al., 2002; DiGirolamo et al., 2001; Grossman et al., 2002; Reuter-Lorenz et al., 2000).

In the Cabeza and colleagues (2002) PET study, older adults with good cognitive skills showed bilateral functioning, while older adults with poorer cognitive skills and younger adults showed lateralized functioning. Further, this was primarily seen on the more demanding memorial tasks. These data indicate that bilateral recruitment during highly demanding cognitive tasks is related to better performance of that task in older adults, while a lack of bilateral recruitment is related to poorer cognitive performance.

Rosen and colleagues (2002) recently found complementary results in a study of semantic encoding. In their study, older adults with initially good memory performance showed left lateralized prefrontal activation, an observation that is similar to that which is seen in younger adults, and greater right prefrontal activation. Older adults with poor initial memory performance had reduced prefrontal activation compared to the other two groups in all areas. These data support the hypothesis of a compensatory process in which we see successful performance in older adults and a lack of biological compensation in less successful older adults.

In summary, neuroimaging studies of healthy older adults have suggested that age-related cognitive declines may be caused by brain changes that result in decreased efficiency in completing cognitive tasks related to hemisphere-specific brain regions. However, recruitment of bilateral brain regions is likely a compensatory strategy during successful aging that mitigates at least some of the cognitive changes that occur as we age. These findings suggest an active process of plasticity of the CNS in adapting to the biological changes that occur and offer an optimistic view of our inherent ability to maintain cognitive function as we age.

Pathological Aging Studies

The clearest and most robust findings in the early functional neuroimaging literature in regards to pathological aging, using PET, have been the consistent findings of the overall reduction of regional cerebral metabolism (hypometabolism), decreases in cerebral perfusion after known pathology, including stroke (Benson et al., 1983; Benson, 1984), and particularly degenerative diseases such as the dementias (Benson, 1982, 1983; Foster et al., 1983; Mazziotta et al., 1987). These findings have been seen both with and without identified structural deficits in the areas of decreased metabolism and have given rise to the view that distant structural deficits can cause functional changes in brain regions that show no structural change but are interconnected to other areas of structural pathology (summarized in Mega et al., 2000; Meyer, Obara, & Muramatsu, 1993). This highlights an important concept in our interpretation of functional deficits seen in aging. That is, when activation deficits are found, particularly in structurally intact areas, we must consider not only the region itself, but its distribution to and from other brain regions. This is not to say that structural and functional deficits do not relate to one another. In fact, in dementing illnesses, structural atrophy is the strongest correlate to decreased metabolic function using PET (Fazeka et al., 1989; Jamieson et al., 1987).

When comparing AD subjects to healthy older adults, the areas of the largest decreases in cerebral perfusion have centered on parietal and temporal association areas (Mega et al., 2000). Similarly, hypometabolism as measured by glucose utilization in PET has been shown in parieto-occipito-temporal association areas in early AD (Benson, 1982; 1983; Ferris et al., 1983; Salmon & Franck, 1989). The fact that these differences are seen in early AD, before other clinical manifestations occur, suggests that functional neuroimaging techniques may be the tools of choice for early identification of dementia (Reiman et al., 1996).

The studies listed earlier have primarily been studies of "resting state" changes in activity. Changes in "active states," when one is engaged in a cognitive task, have been more problematic in dementia because the cognitive impairment that is inherent in this group complicates the interpretation of activity changes. However, in PET and most recently in fMRI, significant strides have been made. Several PET studies by Duara and colleagues (1990, 1992) suggested overall increases in activity in both healthy and AD subjects during verbal and nonverbal memory tasks. Other researchers have provided evidence that healthy older adults show greater overall activity change (Kessler et al., 1991) or larger areas of brain activity (Deutsch & Halsey, 1990; Grady et al., 1993; Woodard et al., 1998) when engaged in cognitive tasks than do AD patients.

fMRI activation studies remain relatively new in the study of dementia. However, Small and colleagues (1999) studied groups of healthy older adults, elders with mild cognitive decline, and AD patients, finding a linear decrease in hippocampal activation across the three groups. Others have found similar results. Burggren, Small, Sabb, and Bookheimer (2002) studied persons with and without the apolipoprotein allele epsiolon 4 (APOE e-4), a genetic risk factor for AD. They found evidence for greater hippocampal region activation in the APOE e-4 carriers than in noncarriers. Johnson and colleagues (2000) have recently focused on the problem of cerebral atrophy in dementing and nondementing older adults. They found that in nondemented older adults, there was no correlation between brain activation during a semantic-decision task of categorical knowledge and cerebral atrophy. However, in mild Alzheimer's disease patients, there was a significant positive correlation with degree of left frontal activation and cerebral atrophy. This has been interpreted as a compensatory recruitment of frontal areas for continued successful engagement in this language-based task in persons suffering from disease-related cerebral atrophy.

Overall, the neuroimaging data on both normal and pathological aging changes suggest a significant change in the brain's role in cognition as we age. Clearly, mechanisms of function change in response to an aging brain, whether due to normal age-related tissue loss or degenerative disease states. However, there appear to be differences both in degree of change and type of change between the two, giving hope that functional neuro-imaging techniques will have greater and greater importance in our ability to differentiate between normal and pathological aging. As an example, Zakzanis, Graham, and Campbell (2003) conducted a meta-analysis of more than 120 structural and functional neuroimaging studies between 1984 and 2000. These studies encompassed more than 5,000 combined AD patients and healthy older adults. They concluded that it is possible to construct "neuroimaging profiles" that include cortical and subcortical neuroanatomic structures, which show promise in reliably separating out AD from non-AD patients.

Cautionary Note

There are a number of limitations that complicate the interpretation of functional imaging data in aging, and these are reviewed by Mega and colleagues (2000). These limitations include deafferentation, which is the loss of neural connections from one area (e.g., subcortical structures) to another (e.g., frontal cortex). Deafferentation confounds the interpretation of findings of metabolic deficit in the absence of concomitant findings of structural deficits. Another limitation is that of partial-volume error, an inherent problem in the averaging techniques for group analysis of functional data. Spatial resolution (e.g., 3-6 mm in PET and SPECT) means that in any given voxel, one is likely to be averaging signals from different components, such as gray matter, white matter, and cerebral spinal fluid (Mazziotta, Phelps, Plummer, & Kuhl, 1981). In aging, particularly the dementias, the common finding of brain tissue atrophy increases this likelihood (increased ventricular size, loss of gray matter). This then increases the likelihood that loss of signal strength will occur as a result of averaging over these disparate tissues. Thus, when we interpret functional imaging data we must be aware of partial volume error.

Recently, there have been a number of analytical techniques that have taken into account partial volume error: the partial volume correction (PVC) methods. These are generally based on segmenting tissue types (e.g., Kollokian, 1996) prior to voxel-based analyses and have been shown to reduce significantly partial volume error (Mega et al., 2000; Müller-Gärtner et al., 1992) with PET data. This has led to more conservative, but likely more reasonable, identification of regional areas of hypometabolism in dementia and aging.

Another area of limitation in interpretation of functional data is the actual way in which data are evaluated. Typically, one either coregisters the functional brain activity collected to regions of interest (ROIs) outlined onto the individual subject's own anatomical images or averages activity within ROIs across subjects onto a common space and then analyzes the data voxel by voxel. Both methods have limitations. In the first case, the ROIs are identified on the anatomical image, but the actual functional activity coregistered is representative of only a single summary statistic representing the entire ROI. This tends to minimize the variability of activity within the entire ROI. Although this is a problem, it can be somewhat overcome by voxel-by-voxel qualitative assessment.

In the second case, averaging across subjects voxel by voxel allows all the data to be utilized but suffers from a reduction of signal intensity when there is variability of anatomy across subjects, as is often the case in older adult brains. Fortunately, several techniques have been developed to minimize these effects, including using Gaussian smoothing, weighted probability maps, and constrained warping of the data at the voxel level to take into account differences in activity around the ROI.

Summary and Speculations of Neuroimaging for Aging, Cognition, and Exercise Research

As can be seen by the information provided so far, neuroimaging has had a significant impact on the way we think about aging. Neuroimaging studies have led to a better understanding of brain changes as we age and how those brain changes affect our cognition. Several results can be summarized. We now know that the brain modestly but consistently loses tissue as it ages and that this affects the way that we process information. We know that tissue changes in pathological disease states look different than those seen in normal aging and that, through high-resolution structural neuroimaging techniques, we may be able to identify these changes early in the process. Further, we know that these pathological changes occur early and that, through functional neuroimaging techniques, we may be able to identify these changes before structural differences are seen.

Regarding the functional changes that occur in the older brain, we now know that metabolic changes occur, primarily reductions in the amount or efficiency of glucose utilization and in cerebral blood flow. We have evidence that these changes are positively associated with cognitive changes in normal aging but particularly in pathological aging processes. One of the important contributions of recent neuroimaging techniques is the support of a model of reduced hemisphere-specialized function as we age. Although at least two hypotheses are possible, evidence suggests that compensatory strategies are activated as we age to minimize the effects of these specialized neuronal regions. This is hopeful news because it indicates a mechanism for dealing with the inevitable loss of integrity of the nervous tissue as we age.

Neuroimaging techniques have opened up a new series of strategies to study the interaction between aging and behavior from a biological perspective. These contributions will only increase as our ability to measure structural and functional brain processes improve. To date, there have been few neuroimaging studies specifically addressing the interplay of aging, cognition, and exercise, which is the primary focus of this book. However, there have been a number of PET studies that have looked at the impact of exercise on brain function. Most of these studies have focused on identifying brain regions modulating cardiovascular responding, but a small number have attempted to address the direct changes of aerobic activity on brain activity (Colcombe et al., 2003; Tashiro et al., 2001).

Critchley and colleagues (2000, 2001) studied the relationship between cognitive states and physiological arousal using PET. In one study (Critchley et al., 2001), they manipulated biofeedback relaxation exercise while undergoing PET scanning, finding increased anterior cingulate and globus pallidus activity during relaxation exercises. This finding suggests an influence of these brain regions on bodily responses. In another study (Critchley et al., 2000), they studied the effects of isometric exercise in healthy adults undergoing PET scanning to determine significant changes in regional cerebral blood flow (rCBF) during states of cardiovascular arousal. They found a significant association with exercise and increased rCBF in several brain regions, including the cerebellar vermis, brain stem and right anterior cingulate; also, there was decreased rCBF in prefrontal and medial temporal regions. Critchley and colleagues (2000) interpreted these results as evidence for the involvement of areas previously implicated in cognitive and emotional behaviors in the representation of increased physiological arousal, making the case that functional organization of the brain for cardiovascular response patterns is associated with activity seen in volitional and emotional behaviors.

Similarly, Thornton and colleagues (2001) used PET to identify neuroanatomical correlates during imagination of exercise under hypnosis, a technique that has been effective in replicating heart rate and ventilation changes akin to actual exercise. They found significant activations in multiple regions including the right dorsolateral prefrontal cortex, supplementary motor area, right premotor area, superolateral sensorimotor areas, and the thalamus and bilaterally in the cerebellum.

Williamson and colleagues (2002) studied real and "imagined" motor activity, that of handgrip. They found that anterior cingulate and insula increased activation during handgrip, but also when "imagined" handgrip occurred in highly hypnotizable participants, indicating these structures' role in the central modulation of cardiovascular responses. In a more direct assessment of the influence of exercise on brain activity, Tashiro and colleagues (2001) used PET to assess glucose metabolism in the brain and contrasted a group of healthy younger adults following running several kilometers to a resting control group. They found that running correlated with increased glucose uptake in the temporoparietal association cortex, occipital cortex, premotor cortex, and the cerebellar vermis. Greatest increases were observed in the temporoparietal association cortex; also, the primary sensorimotor cortex was higher in areas for leg control compared to upper-body control. Data indicate the sensitivity of functional neuroimaging in identifying immediate metabolic changes as a consequence of exercise.

In one of the few studies actually using neuroimaging techniques to assess the effects of exercise in older adults, Colcombe and colleagues (2003) took high-resolution structural MRI scans of a substantial number of older adults ($n = 55$), segmented them for volumetric assessment, and compared these markers to age and aerobic fitness as well as to several other health markers. Their study indicated, as expected, that there are age-related declines in tissue density and volume in multiple brain regions. However, they also found a relationship between level of aerobic fitness and reduced density and volume loss. This is one of the first studies to use neuroimaging techniques to verify exercise benefits in older adults beyond simple cardiovascular improvement.

Although small in number, the studies discussed earlier indicate that brain regions modulating physiological arousal, such as exercise, can be identified using functional neuroimaging techniques. In combination with the large amount of data on cognitive neuroimaging in aging research, these studies give us a sense of what realizations might result from studies integrating aging, cognition, and exercise. Neuroimaging, particularly functional neuroimaging, appears able to give us heretofore unrealized information regarding the relationship between exercise and brain function. This, in turn, suggests that these techniques hold promise in being able to explicate some of the most difficult questions regarding the impact of exercise on cognitive loss, change, and plasticity in older adults. At least one study has used these techniques specific to aging and exercise (Colcombe et al., 2003).

Additionally, a recent proposal of using functional neuroimaging techniques to assess the combined influence of exercise on cognition in older adults has been put forth (Kramer, Colcombe, Erickson, et al., 2002). Relying on studies such as those reviewed earlier and the extant animal literature indicating neurotransmitter and even morphological brain changes following aerobic exercise, Kramer and colleagues established a proposition. They suggested that functional neuroimaging techniques can play an important role in human fitness intervention studies by providing a window into the functional changes that occur in real time in the brain at pre- and postfitness training. They go on to advocate aggressive research expansion using these techniques. Proposals such as this will likely help us overcome the difficulties in observing subtle cognitive change that are a result of exercise or in observing the biochemical changes (e.g., increased blood flow) that may occur as a result of exercise, allowing for the quantification and visualization of these changes using functional neuroimaging techniques.

CHAPTER 11

Issues of Aging, Physical Activity, Cognition, and Putative Mechanisms for a Relationship: A Discussion

Waneen W. Spirduso, EdD

In 1980, I published a review paper "Physical Fitness, Aging, and Psychomotor Speed: A Review," and today I am pondering how much we have learned about health, fitness, and cognition in 25 years. In those early years of this research topic, it was very clear that many cognitive processes suffered when health was poor and pathology was present. But questioning whether improved health and fitness might provide additional benefits to the cognitive function of older adults was considered somewhat radical. In fact, those types of research questions in the late 1970s garnered more than their fair share of doubt and derision. Since that time, hundreds of papers have been published on some aspect of this proposed relationship, either in terms of behavioral outcomes or putative mechanisms to explain such a relationship. We do not yet have definitive answers regarding this topic, but we have made much progress in elucidating the issues and problems of research and in identifying possible mechanisms by which activity may affect cognitive function. This chapter summarizes and comments on the issues and major questions that repeatedly emerged throughout our discussions at the Advanced Research Workshop held at St. Simon's Island, Georgiz in 2002.

Our general impression is that physical activity in some form is related to cognitive function, but many issues are unresolved. These issues can be summarized as (a) the quandary surrounding physical activity, (b) the specifics of cognition, (c) the likely target of beneficial effects of physical activity, (d) the strength of the relationship, (e) whether physical activity effects are nonadditive for individuals of different ages, (f) the role of individual differences, and (g) the potent role of research design in the outcomes of this type of research. The following discussion is based on the assumption that the reader has read the papers in the previous section.

What Type of Physical Activity Influences Cognition?

If physical movement in some form is related to cognition in such a way that it either maintains or improves cognitive function, what type of movement is required to effect this outcome? At present, researchers use the terms physical activity, exercise, aerobic training, and lifestyle activity almost interchangeably with little attention to a definition. Dependent variables in these studies are many times quite different, depending on their implicit definition of movement activity. As long as this situation remains, it will be difficult to compare the results of research studies. Dishman (chapter 6) and Cress (chapter 7) provided some guidelines in measuring activities and physical performances that could be used as common metrics to quantify for comparison sake the levels of activities, training, and aerobic fitness.

The type of movement necessary will probably depend on whatever turn out to be the mechanisms that support such a relationship. If moderate arousal levels and neural stimulation or merely the absence of cerebrovascular disease can maintain cognition, then moderate levels of physical activity, that is, an avoidance of sedentary behavior by doing almost any type of movement would be sufficient. If increased cerebral blood flow and oxygen delivery is linearly or curvilinearly related to cognitive function, then exercise training that increases aerobic capacity would be requisite. But what does the brain need to function efficiently? Does it require a minimum level of underlying substrate, above which additional oxygen delivery or other blood chemistry levels and interactions have little additional effect? In other words, is there a *threshold effect*, so that if old adults (or others with disease states) fall below this threshold, cognition is impaired? Is there a *cognitive reserve* that could be quantified, that is, the distance of cognitive function from threshold, or minimum, that impairs performance? Can exercise be thought of as a mechanism, along with others, that optimizes the brain biochemical milieu so that it can function efficiently?

Activities that make large demands cognitively may influence cognition more than repetitive, cyclic activities. Tai chi (chapter 7) is an example of a physical activity that is thought to require intense concentration and other cognitive goals throughout the movement. Similarly, a computerized exercise dance instrumentation, which is very popular in Japan, is said to require intense mental focus, executive function, and high-level physical strength and endurance in order to perform it. Might it be expected that habitual performance of physical activities that have a high "cognitive load" benefit cognition more than a lifetime of jogging or walking?

These are critical questions that need to be answered in order to consolidate training and activity regimens related to cognitive maintenance in older adults. Dustman and White (chapter 4) and Holmes (chapter 5) provided cogent reviews on the impact of exercise on basic functional properties of the brain. Information contained in these chapters would be helpful to form hypotheses relating to these questions.

Specifics of Cognition

As is the case with physical movement, the term *cognition* has many times been used very loosely to mean brain or mental function, and has not been defined very carefully. When it is defined specifically, the range of cognitive functions that have been investigated in physical activity–cognition studies is very broad. Cognitive supportive functions are thought to be attention (resource allocation), working memory, processing speed, motor output, and perceptual processes (also see reviews in chapter 1, Chodzko-Zajko, and chapter 2, Tomporowski). Some basic cognitive operations are memory, association, comparison, abstract reasoning, spatial ability, and synthesis. Higher-order cognitive processes proposed are executive control (planning, scheduling, coordination, inhibition) and the broader constructs of primary mental abilities and intelligence. Most of these functions can be assessed at different levels of effort, from very simple to very complex tests. The challenge to synthesizers of the physical activity–cognition research literature is to make sense of results from studies that vary widely across both domains: the focus on different aspects of cognition and the use of test instruments that make different demands along the simple–complex dimension.

In chapter 3, Poon and Harrington attempted such a synthesis by examining the utility of different types of measures in supporting different postulated cognitive mechanisms in aging and fitness. From this perspective, the variety of cognitive measures employed in the literature might not be as haphazard as it seemed. For example, in studies that purported to evaluate the theories of attention resource reduction, the researchers tended to employ tasks that varied in the amount of effort and attention required. Researchers who examined the theories of frontal system deficit tended to employ tasks varying in levels of central executive control. Those who examined the general decrement theories had employed a gamut of tasks in order to access the characteristics of the overall information processor. It is important to note that the selection of cognitive tasks needs to be driven by the research question.

Proposed Cognitive Targets of Physical Activity Effects

The early researchers of exercise and cognition focused on processing speed in reaction-time paradigms using simple reaction time that required only one stimulus interpretation, and choice reaction time that required different reactions to two or more stimuli. They found that greater relationships with fitness were found with choice than with simple reaction time. It was proposed that complex processing of stimuli, being more sensitive to aging, was also more affected by health and fitness. This reasoning developed into the hypothesis that the cognitive functions that demand greater allocation of resources would also reflect a greater relationship with fitness levels. Effortful tasks, which required more resource management, were thought to be influenced more by fitness than noneffortful tasks. Thus, studies were conducted with time-sharing tasks and tasks that stressed attention mechanisms. Problems arose, however, because some studies failed to find cognitive differences in fitness groups, whether the dependent variable was complex reaction time or tasks that stressed resource allocation. In fact, we have lived through two decades in which contradictory results from studies of fitness–cognition relationships can be found in variables as diverse as working memory, perceptual processes, association, spatial ability, and motor output.

This state of affairs did not appear to be changing, until results published from A.F. Kramer's laboratory (Colcombe & Kramer, 2003) predicted that an exercise intervention would influence cognitive tasks requiring executive control more than it would affect single-operation tasks that stressed functions such as visual search, spatial attention, pursuit rotor, working memory, or perceptual comparisons. This hypothesis is especially appealing because executive control has been identified through magnetic resonance imaging as associated with prefrontal and frontal regions of the brain and these regions are thought to age at a disproportionately faster rate than other brain regions. In addition, differential circulatory decline in the frontal and prefrontal lobes would provide a mechanism to explain beneficial effects of fitness on executive control function. Hall, Smith, and Keele (2001) analyzed *post hoc* the cognitive tasks of Hawkins, Kramer, and Capaldi (1992) and of Abourezk and Toole (1995) and found these to fall within the criteria for tests of executive control. All three of these studies were consistent in finding that executive control but not other cognitive operations were affected by an exercise intervention. It is our understanding that Kramer and his colleagues are continuing to test this hypothesis and are utilizing functional MRI to determine cerebral blood flow relationships with cognitive performance. These findings should generate quite a lot of excitement in this area. A good summary of the rationale for fitness affecting executive control can be found in the review by Hawkins, Kramer, and Capaldi (1992).

How Strong Is the Relationship Between Exercise and Physical Activity and Aging?

Several lines of research suggest that the relationship is robust. Animal research provides the strongest evidence. Holmes (chapter 5) suggests that the facts that (a) both movement activation and motivation mechanisms reside in the basal ganglia, (b) attention, motivation, and movement mechanisms appear together in the locus coeruleus, and (c) both of these areas are influenced by exercise provides a strong argument that cognition and movement are related. Many investigators have shown that physical activity and motor learning directly affect neurotransmitter systems in the basal ganglia. Exercise training has also been shown to profoundly improve results on tests of performance and learning in animals. These studies should not be overlooked in the analysis of the physical activity–cognition relationship.

Moving from the study of animal models to human performance has been much more problematic. Cross-sectional studies provide the next strongest evidence to support an activity–cognition linkage. In these studies, older adults who are healthier and have higher levels of physical fitness have almost universally performed better on cognitive tests than their unhealthy and unfit counterparts. Furthermore, Poon and Harrington (chapter 3) in a meta-analysis of 10 studies showed that the magnitude of difference between the active and inactive older groups was linearly related to the cognitive-task demands, being almost nonexistent for minimal cognitive processing and almost 50 to 100 percent larger for high demands for processing. However, cross-sectional studies are always plagued with the flaw that a variety of relevant individual differences in characteristics might not have been adequately controlled between the fit and less fit groups. For example, the people in exercise groups and cohorts may have been genetically predisposed to higher cognitive function throughout their life, rather than reflecting the benefits of an exercise intervention in the study at hand. Issues relating to individual differences as well as direct and indirect effects of exercise through mediating mechanisms need to be better explicated. An experimental study in which physical activity and exercise intervenes between pre- and postcognitive testing would be more convincing. However, as noted in chapters 1 (Chodzko-Zajko) and chapter 2 (Tomporowski), these studies have not provided clear-cut results. Nevertheless, the consistency in findings comparing the cognitive performances between the fit and less fit older adults (see chapter 2) indicates that this finding is robust.

Exercise intervention studies of humans, however, have generally been disappointing. Many of these experimental researchers found no differences between physically active and nonactive groups on cognitive assessments, and those who did find differences reported that the effects were small. However, some of the most quoted of these intervention studies have had research design problems. Research on the effects of moderating and mediating mechanisms between exercise and activity and cognition is therefore much needed prior to large-scale studies of intervention.

A question that continues to surface regarding the physical activity effect is whether there is a threshold effect of physical activity, or, as someone in the audience always asks after a discussion of this subject, "What is the smallest amount of exercise I can get away with and still keep my mind functioning as well as it always has?" This will be an important question to answer in the future, but we do not have the answer now.

Another question related to the amount of activity necessary to effect a change in cognition is, "What if the overall benefit of activity on cognition turns out to be a very small percentage? What if physical activity under the best of conditions for a long duration only enhances cognition 5 or 10 percent? Or, what if the benefit is only the maintenance of existing cognitive efficiency, that is, a deceleration of decline rather than an improvement in function?" Arguments can be made that either of these situations is of value. Gains in function are relative as well as absolute. A 5 percent gain in leg strength may provide almost no visible gain in speed performance for an athlete, but would mean the difference between being able to walk or not walk for an 85-year-old woman. A 5 percent gain in processing speed in an older man could mean the difference between being hit by a car or passing safely across a street. Similarly, for elderly adults who wish desperately to retain as much cognitive processing efficiency as possible for as long as possible, simply maintaining useful function to live independently is extremely valuable. An analogy might be made here with results from cognition enhancing drug studies in Alzheimer's disease (AD). Four drugs had been approved by the Food and Drug Administration (FDA) for treatment of cognitive dysfunction associated with AD. Studies show that the facilitative effect is about 5 percent and no more than 10 percent. However, family members and clinical staff reported a noticeable difference in everyday cognition with this effect size. From this perspective, a 5 percent increase in cognitive performance can make a difference in the everyday life of older adults.

Finally, the research community has expressed the desire that studies could eventually determine whether a dose-response relationship exists between physical activity intensity and duration and cognitive benefits. Our conclusion was that we are still very much in a framework of uncertainty as to the nature and extent of an activity–cognition relationship, and the establishment of a dose-response relationship seems very far down the experimental road.

Comments and Questions About Mechanisms

A review of chapters in this volume suggests that mechanisms proposed to explain a physical activity–cognition relationship can be grouped into two categories: those that explain the relationship by cognitive or behavioral mechanisms (see chapters 1 through 3) and those that explain the relationship by physiological or neurobiological mechanisms (see chapters 4 and 5). These chapters provide excellent reviews to form interdisciplinary research questions and research.

What is the relationship between direct and indirect effects of exercise on cognition?   Physical activity may influence cognitive function either directly by affecting brain structure and function, indirectly by affecting other factors known to influence brain structure and function, or by a combination of direct and indirect influences. Some indirect influences may be through the role of exercise in improving such factors as sleep, lipid profiles, hypertension, reduction of comorbidities, reduction of anxiety and depression, and the amelioration of pain.

Can we eventually develop a temporal template that describes when different potential mechanisms are developed by physical activity?   For example, several physiological responses have been reported to change very quickly with an acute bout of exercise: cerebral blood flow, reversal of hypoxia, metabolic changes, local control of glucose, and expression of the intermediate early gene c-fos. Other proposed mechanisms such as retrograde and anterograde transport of trophic factors and beneficial effects on depressive systems are thought to occur after three or four weeks of vigorous physical activity. Still others have been proposed as long-term changes related to exercise: lowered resting heart rate, monamine desensitization and upregulation, neural sprouting, axonal regeneration, synaptogenesis, and trophic changes.

How likely is it that the chronic effects of exercise are really the repeated effects of acute exercise done every day?   Tomporowski (chapter 2) points out that at present no studies are available in which the investigators have examined "the impact of individual exercise bouts that take place in the context of long-term training." It would be particularly important to study neurohormonal or neurotrophic mechanisms in a design where acute bouts are experienced on a regular basis, paralleled by assessments of cognition as a dependent variable and interrupted and restarted in different groups at different times and for different lengths of time. Follow-up measures would be crucial in comparing acute to chronic effects.

How important are new innovations in neurobiological and neurophysiological measures in advancing this field of exercise and cognition?   McCully and Bhambhani (chapter 9) and Miller (chapter 10) provided examples of noninvasive techniques that can directly test several key hypotheses of exercise and cognition relating to blood flow and frontal system mechanisms. These new technologies promise to produce great strides in our understanding of this topic in the near future.

Noncognitive Factors
Strongly Influence Cognition

A multitude of noncognitive factors other than exercise affect cognition. Examples are sleep, pain, anxiety and depression, adiposity, lipid profiles, blood chemistry, blood pressure, medications, smoking, alcohol, comorbidities, social effects, and many others. O'Connor (chapter 8) points out that neuropsychological impairment occurs in people who experience pain, and the more intense the pain, the greater the impairment seen. Physical activity affects many of these noncognitive factors in predominantly positive ways but also in some negative ways. Physical activity can reduce osteoporotic and osteoarthritic pain and can improve sleep (King et al., 1997). Exercise can contribute to the reduction of depressive symptoms, but it also may produce fatigue or cause or aggravate pain in the joints. Research studies of exercise and cognition in the future must be designed so that the direct effects of these factors, the indirect effects of exercise on these factors, and their interactions can be identified.

Cognitive Function
Influences Physical Function

We have been focusing on the potential influences of physical activity and exercise on cognitive function. Yet, it is becoming more and more apparent that the reverse is operative: Impaired cognition negatively affects physical function. When a cognitive task is introduced as a secondary task to be executed during a challenge to maintain balance in the face of a perturbation, muscular response to the perturbation is not slower, but the amplitude is less (Rankin, Woollacot, Shumway-Cook, & Brown, 2000). Thus, although older adults may respond as quickly to a perturbation in their base of support while counting backward by threes as they do when not counting, the amount of response may not be adequate to prevent a fall.

It has been well documented that cognitive capacity is associated with activities of daily living and instrumental activities of daily living. Carlson and colleagues (1999) have pointed out that executive attention is important in mediating the onset and progression of physical function decline. Tinetti, Speechley, and Ginter (1988) found that cognitive impairment in community dwellers was the largest contributor to falls. Cognitive impairment presents methodological problems as well: It also affects the accuracy of self-report of physical function (Carlson et al., 1999). Finally, intact cognition is necessary to initiate an exercise or physical activity program, to plan it, and to maintain it.

Next Steps

All of the researchers who participated in the advanced research workshop (and whose reviews make up this volume) continually brought up their observations that many factors influence cognition: individual differences, environmental factors, health status, self-esteem, and many others. A clear direction emerged from the reviews published in this volume: To obtain meaningful cognitive change with exercise intervention, we need to address all substantive and ecological-related factors that can affect cognition. Thus, our next volume addresses the mediating mechanisms between activity and fitness and cognitive functioning. First, we provide a discussion of the nature of a mediator and how it might be quantified. We then suggest that three large categories of mediators affect cognition: *physical resources* (energy and fatigue, sleep effectiveness, and nutritional status), *disease states* (hypertension, diabetes, cardiovascular and cerebrovascular status, and chronic obstruction and pulmonary disease), and *mental resources* (self-efficacy, chronic stress, and depression). The review of how physical activity might influence these resources, which in turn may mediate (either negatively or positively) certain types of cognitive function, is the theme of volume 2. The goals of volume 2 are threefold: To (1) review research results to identify and validate paths, direct and indirect, by which exercise and physical activities can influence cognition; (2) suggest mediators that most potently interact with exercise, cognition, and aging; and finally (3) recommend research directions that could consolidate these mechanisms in future research designs.

REFERENCES

Abourezk, T. (1989). The effects of regular aerobic exercise on short-term memory efficiency in the older adult. In A.C. Ostrow (Ed.), *Aging and motor behavior* (pp. 105-113). Indianapolis: Benchmark Press.

Abourezk, T., & Toole, T. (1995). Effect of task complexity on the relationship between physical fitness and reaction time in older women. *Journal of Aging & Physical Activity, 3,* 251-260.

Ades, P.A., Waldmann, M.L., & Gillespie, C. (1995). A controlled trial of exercise training in older coronary patients. *Journal of Gerontology: Biological Sciences & Medical Sciences, 50A(1),* M7-M11.

Ahto, M., Isoaho, R., Puolijoki, H., Laippala, P., Sulkava, R., & Kivela, S.L. (1999). Cognitive impairment among elderly coronary heart disease patients. *Gerontology, 45(2),* 87-95.

Ajmani, R.S., Metter, E.J., Jaykumar, R., Ingram, D.K., Spangler, E.L., Abugo, O.O., et al. (2000). Hemodynamic changes during aging associated with cerebral blood flow and impaired cognitive function. *Neurobiology of Aging, 21,* 257-269.

Albert, M.S., & Kaplan, E. (1980). Organic implications of neuropsychological deficits in the elderly. In L.W. Poon, J.L. Fozard, L.S. Cermak, D. Arenberg, & L.W. Thompson (Eds.), *New direction in memory and aging.* Mahwah, NJ: Lawrence Erlbaum.

Altar, C.A. (1999). Neurotrophins and depression. *Trends in Pharmacological Sciences, 20,* 59-61.

Anderson, B.J., Rapp, D.N., Baek, D.H., McCloskey, D.P., Coburn-Litvak, P.S., & Robinson, J.K. (2000). Exercise influences spatial learning in the radial arm maze. *Physiology & Behavior, 70,* 425-429.

Anderson, N.D., Iidaka, T., McIntosh, A.R., Kapur, S., Cabeza, R., & Craik, F.I.M. (2000). The effects of divided attention on encoding- and retrieval-related brain activity: A PET study of younger and older adults. *Journal of Cognitive Neuroscience, 12,* 775-792.

Andersson, H.I., Ejlertsson, G., Leden, I., & Rosenberg, C. (1993). Chronic pain in a geographically defined general population: Studies of differences in age, gender, social class, and pain localization. *Clinical Journal of Pain, 9,* 174-82.

Aniansson A., Grimby G., Nygaard E., & Saltin B. (1980). Muscle fiber composition and fiber area in various age groups. *Muscle & Nerve,* May/June, 271-273.

Arida, R.M., Scorza, F.A., dos Santos, N.F., Peres, C.A., & Cavalheiro, E.A. (1999). Effect of physical activity on seizure occurrence in a model of temporal lobe epilepsy in rats. *Epilepsy Research, 37,* 45-52.

References

Armstrong S., Sloan, S., Turner, M., et al. (2001). National blueprint: Increasing physical activity among adults age 50 and older. *Journal of Aging & Physical Activity, 9,* 5-13.

Ashburner, J., & Friston, K.J. (2000). Voxel-based morphometry—The methods. *Neuroimage, 11,* 805-821.

Åstrand, P.-O. (1988). From exercise physiology to preventive medicine. *Annals of Clinical Research, 20,* 10-17.

Åstrand, P.-O. (1992). Physical activity and fitness. *American Journal of Clinical Nutrition, 55,* 1231S-1236S.

Åstrand, P.-O. (1994). Physical activity and fitness: Evolutionary perspective and trends for the future. In C. Bouchard, R.J. Shephard, & T. Stephens (Eds.), *Physical activity, fitness, and health: International proceedings and consensus statement.* (pp. 98-105). Champaign, IL: Human Kinetics.

Åstrand, P.-O., & Rodahl, K. (1986). Our biologic heritage. In P.-O. Åstrand, & K. Rodahl (Eds.), *Textbook of work physiology* (pp. 1-11). New York: McGraw-Hill.

Azmitia, E.C., & Whitaker-Azmitia, P.M. (1995). Anatomy, cell biology, and plasticity of the serotonergic system. In F.E. Bloom, & D.J. Kupfer (Eds.), *Psychopharmacology: The fourth generation of progress.* (pp. 443-449). New York: Raven Press.

Baker, A.P. (1999). The Raymond Pearl memorial lecture: The eternal triangle-genes, phenotype, and the environment. *American Journal of Human Biology, 9,* 93-101.

Baltes, P.B., & Lindenberger, U. (1997). Emergence of a powerful connection between sensory and cognitive functions across the adult life span: A new window to the study of cognitive aging? *Psychology and Aging, 12,* 12-21.

Barlow, J.S. (1993). *The electroencephalogram: Its patterns and origins.* Cambridge, MA: MIT Press.

Bassett, D.R. (2000). Validity and reliability issues in objective monitoring of physical activity. *Research Quarterly for Exercise & Sport, 71,* 30-36.

Bassett, D.R., Ainsworth, B.E., Leggett, S.R., Mathien, C.A., Main, J.A., Hunter, D.C., & Duncan, G.E. (1996). Accuracy of five electronic pedometers for measuring distance walked. *Medicine & Science in Sports & Exercise, 28,* 1071-1077.

Bassey, E.J., Fiatarone, M.A, O'Neil, E.F., Kelly, M., & Evans, W.J. (1992). Leg extensor power and functional performance in very old men and women. *Clinical Science, 82,* 321-327.

Baylor, A.M., & Spirduso, W.W. (1988). Systematic aerobic exercise and components of reaction time in older women. *Journal of Gerontology:Psychological Sciences, 43*(5), 121-126.

Beck, E.C. (1975). Electrophysiology and behavior. *Annual Review of Psychology, 26,* 233-262.

Belardinelli, R., Barstow, T., Porszasz, J., & Wasserman, K. (1995). Changes in muscle O_2 saturation with incremental exercise measured with near infrared spectroscopy. *European Journal of Applied Physiology & Occupational Health, 70,* 487-492.

References

Benson, D.F. (1982). Cerebral metabolism in aging and dementia. *Neurology and Neurosurgery Update Series, 3,* 1-8.

Benson, D.F. (1983). Alterations in glucose metabolism in Alzheimer's disease. In *Biological aspects of Alzheimer's disease* (Banbury Report 15). (pp. 309-315). Cold Spring Harbor, NY: Cold Spring Harbor Laboratory Press.

Benson, D.F., (1984). Positron emission tomography in aphasia. *Seminars in Neurology, 4,* 169-173.

Benson, D.F., Kuhl, D.E., Hawkins, R.A., Phelps, M.E., Cummings, J.L., & Tsay, S.Y. (1983). The fluorodexyglucose ^{18}F scan in Alzheimer's disease and multi-infarct dementia. *Archives of Neurology, 40,* 711-714.

Benvenuti, F., Ferrucci, L., Guralnik, J.M., Gangemi, S., & Baroni, A. (1995). Foot pain and disability in older persons: An epidemiologic survey. *Journal of the American Geriatrics Society, 43(5),* 479-484.

Berchtold, N.C., Kesslak, J.P., Pike, C.J., Adlard, P.A., & Cotman, C.W. (2001). Estrogen and exercise interact to regulate brain-derived neurotrophic factor mRNA and protein expression in the hippocampus. *European Journal of Neuroscience, 14,* 1992-2002.

Berger, B.G., & Hecht, L.M. (1990). Exercise, aging and psychological well-being: The mind-body question. In A.C. Ostrow (Ed.), *Aging and motor behavior* (pp. 307-323). Indianapolis: Benchmark Press.

Berger, H. (1969). On the electroencephalogram of man. The fourteen original reports on the human electroencephalogram. (P. Gloor, Trans., Ed.). *Electroencephalography & Clinical Neuropsychology, (Suppl. 28).*

Berridge, K.C., & Robinson, T.E. (1998). What is the role of dopamine in reward: Hedonic impact, reward learning, or incentive salience? *Brain Research Reviews, 28,* 309-369.

Bihan, D. (1994). Microcirculation and perfusion. In R. Gillies (Ed.), *NMR in physiology and biomedicine* (pp. 43-54). San Diego: Academic Press.

Binder, E.F., Schenkman, K.B., Ehsani, A.A., Steger-May, K., Brown, M., Sinacore, D.R., Yarasheski, K.E., & Halloszy, J.O. (2002). Effects of exercise training on frailty in community-dwelling older adults: Results of a randomized, controlled trial. *Journal of the American Geriatrics Society, 50,* 1921-1928.

Binder, E.F., Storandt, M., & Birge, S.J. (1999). The relation between psychometric test performance and physical performance in older adults. *Journal of Gerontology: Medical Sciences, 54A(8),* M428-M432.

Birren, J.E. (1965). Age changes in speed of behavior: Its central nature and physiological correlates. In A.T. Welford & J.E. Birren (Eds.), *Behavior, aging and the nervous system* (pp. 191-216). Springfield, IL: Thomas.

Bixler, E.O., Kales, A., Soldatos, C. R., Kales, J.D., & Healey, S. (1979). Prevalence of sleep disorders in the Los Angeles metropolitan area. *American Journal of Psychiatry, 136(10),* 1257-1262.

Black, A.E. (1996). Physical activity levels from a meta-analysis of doubly labeled water studies for validating energy intake as measured by dietary assessment. *Nutrition Review, 54(6),* 170-174.

References

Black, J.E. (1998). How a child builds its brain: Some lessons from animal studies of neural plasticity. *Preventive Medicine, 27,* 168-171.

Blatter, D.D, Bigler, E.D., Gale, S.D., Johnson, S.C., Anderson, C.V., Burnett, B.M., et al. (1995). Quantitative volumetric analysis of brain MR: Normative database spanning 5 decades of life. *American Journal of Neuroradiology, 16,* 241-251.

Blesa, R., Mohr, E., Miletich, R.S., Randolph, C., Hildebrand, K., Sampson, M., & Chase, T.N. (1997). Changes in cerebral glucose metabolism with normal aging. *European Journal of Neurology, 4,* 8-14.

Bliwise, D.L. (1993). Sleep in normal aging and dementia. *Sleep, 16(1),* 40-81.

Bliwise, D.L., King, A.C., Harris, R.B., & Haskell, W.L. (1992). Prevalence of self-reported poor sleep in a healthy population aged 50-65. *Social Science and Medicine, 34(1),* 49-55.

Bloch, G.J., Butler, P.C., Eckersell, C.B., & Mills, R.H. (1998). Gonadal steroid-dependent GAL-IR cells within the medial preoptic nucleus and the stimulatory effect of GAL within the MPN on sexual behaviors. In Galanin Basic Research and Therapeutic Implications. *Annals of the New York Academy of Sciences, 863,* 188-205.

Bloom, F.E., Lazerson, A., & Hofstadter, L. (1985). *Brain, mind, and behavior.* New York: W.H. Freeman.

Blumenthal, J.A., Babyak, M.A., Moore, K.A., Craighead, W.E., Herman, S., Khatri, P., Waugh, R., Napolitano, M.A., Forman, L.M., Appelbaum, M., Doraiswamy, P.M., & Krishnan, K.R. (1999). Effects of exercise training on older patients with major depression. *Archives of Internal Medicine, 159(19),* 2349-2356.

Blumenthal, J.A., Emery, C.F., Madden, D.J., George, L.K., Coleman, R.E., Riddle, M.W., McKee, D.C., Reasoner, J., & Williams, R.S. (1989). Cardiovascular and behavioral effects of aerobic exercise training in healthy older men and women. *Journal of Gerontology: Medical Science, 44(5),* M147-M157.

Blumenthal, J.A., Emery, C.F., Madden, D.J., Schniebolk, S., Walsh-Riddle, M., George, L.K., McKee, D.C., Higginbotham, M.B., Cobb, F.R., & Coleman, R.E. (1991). Long-term effects of exercise on psychological functioning in older men and women. *Journal of Gerontology: Psychological Sciences, 46,* P352-P361.

Blumenthal, J.A., & Madden, D.J. (1988). Effects of aerobic exercise training, age, and physical fitness on memory-search performance. *Psychology & Aging, 3,* 280-285.

Bohannon, A.D., Fillenbaum, G.G., Pieper, C.F., Hanlon, J.T., & Blazer, D.G. (2002). Relationship of race/ethnicity and blood pressure to change in cognitive function. *Journal of the American Geriatrics Society, 50(3),* 424-429.

Booth, F.W., Chakravarthy, M.V., Gordon, S.E., & Spangenburg, E.E. (2002). Waging war on physical inactivity: Using modern molecular ammunition against an ancient enemy. *Journal of Applied Physiology, 93(1),* 3-30.

Booyens, J., & Hervey, G.R. (1960). The pulse rate as a means of measuring metabolic rate in man. *Canadian Journal of Biochemical Physiology, 38,* 1301.

Bortolotto, L., Hanon, O., Franconi, G., Boutouyrie, P., Legrain, S., & Girerd, X. (1999). The aging process modifies the distensibility of elastic but not muscular arteries. *Hypertension, 34,* 889-892.

References

Bortz, W.M. (1989). Redefining human aging. *Journal of the American Geriatrics Society, 37,* 1092-1096.

Bouchard, C., Shephard, R.J., & Stephens, T. (Eds.). (1994). *Physical activity, fitness, and health: Consensus statement.* Champaign, IL: Human Kinetics.

Boutcher, S.H. (2000). Cognitive performance, fitness, and ageing. In S.J.H. Biddle, K.R. Fox, & S.H. Boutcher (Eds.), *Physical activity and psychological well-being* (pp. 118-129). New York: Routledge.

Bowles, N.L., Obler, L.K., & Poon, L.W. (1989). Aging and word retrieval: Naturalistic, clinical, and laboratory data. In L.W. Poon, D.C. Rubin, et al. (Eds.), *Everyday cognition in adulthood and late life* (xii, pp. 244-264). New York: Cambridge University Press.

Brandt, E.N., Jr., & Pope, A.M. (1997). *Enabling America: Assessing the role of rehabilitation science and engineering.* Washington, D.C.: National Academy Press.

Brassington, G.S., & Hicks, R.A. (1995). Aerobic exercise and self-reported sleep quality in elderly individuals. *Journal of Aging & Physical Activity, 3(2),* 120-134.

Brassington, G.S., King, A.C., & Bliwise, D.L. (2000). Sleep problems as a risk factor for falls in a sample of community-dwelling adults aged 64-99 years. *Journal of the American Geriatrics Society, 48(10),* 1234-1240.

Brochu, M., Savage, P., Lee, M., Cress, M.E., Poehlman, E.T., Dee, J., Tischler, M., & Ades, P.A. (2002). Resistance training in older women with coronary heart disease: A randomized controlled trial. *Journal of Applied Physiology, 92,* 672-678.

Brouha L., Smith, P.E., Jr. (1958). Energy expenditure of motions [Abstract]. *Federation Proceedings of the American Society for Experimental Biology, 17,* 20.

Brown, B.S., & Van Huss, W. (1973). Exercise and rat brain catecholamines. *Journal of Applied Physiology, 34,* 664-669.

Brown, S.C., Glass, J.M., & Park, D.C. (2002). The relationship of pain and depression to cognitive function in rheumatoid arthritis patients. *Pain, 96(3),* 279-84.

Brun, A., & Englund, E. (1981). Regional pattern of degeneration in Alzheimer disease: Neuronal loss and histopathological grading. *Histopathology, 5,* 549-564.

Buchner, D.M., Cress, M.E., Esselman, P.C., Margherita, A.J., deLateur, B.J., Campbell, A.J., & Wagner, E.H. (1996). Factors associated with changes in gait speed in older adults. *Journal of Gerontology: Medical Sciences, 51A(6),* M297-M302.

Buchner, D.M., Guralnik, J.M., & Cress, M.E. (1995). The clinical assessment of gait, balance, and mobility in older adults. In L. Z. Rubenstein, D. Wieland, & R. Bernabei (Eds.), *Geriatric assessment technology: The state of the art* (pp. 75-89). Milan, Italy: Kurtis.

Buchner, K., Meixensberger, J., Dings, J., & Roosen, K. (2000). Near-infrared spectroscopy: Not useful to monitor cerebral oxgyenation after severe brain injury. *Zentralblatt für Neurochirurgi, 61,* 69-73.

Burggren, A.C., Small, G.W., Sabb, F.W., & Bookheimer, S.Y. (2002). Specificity of brain activation patterns in people at genetic risk for Alzheimer disease. *American Journal of Geriatric Psychiatry, 10,* 44-51.

Bush, G., Luu, P., & Posner, M.I. (2000). Cognitive and emotional influences in anterior cingulate cortex. *Trends in Cognitive Science, 4(6)*, 215-222.

Caballero, A., Arora, S., Saouaf, R., Lim, S., Smakowski, P., Park, J., King, G., LoGerfo, F., Horton, E., & Veves, A. (1999). Microvascular and macrovascular reactivity is reduced in subjects at risk for type 2 diabetes. *Diabetes, 48*, 1856-1862.

Cabeza, R. (2001). Cognitive neuroscience of aging: Contributions of functional neuroimaging. *Scandinavian Journal of Psychology, 42*, 277-286.

Cabeza, R. (2002). Hemispheric asymmetry reduction in old adults: The HAROLD Model. *Psychology & Aging, 17*, 85-100.

Cabeza, R., Anderson, N.D., Locantore, J.K., & McIntosh, A.R. (2002). Aging gracefully: Compensatory brain activity in high-performing older adults. *NeuroImage, 17*, 1394-1402.

Cabeza, R., Grady, C.L., Nyberg, L., McIntosh, A.R., Tulving, E., Kapur, S., Jennings, J.M., Houle, S., & Craik, F.I.M. (1997). Age-related differences in neural activity during memory encoding and retrieval: A positron emission tomography study. *Journal of Neuroscience, 17*, 391-400.

Camacho, T.C., Roberts, R.E., Lazarus, N.B., Kaplan, G.A., & Cohen, R.D. (1991). Physical activity and depression: Evidence from the Alameda County Study. *American Journal of Epidemiology, 134(2)*, 220-231.

Cardillo, C., Kilcoyne, C., Cannon, R., & Panza, J. (1999). Attenuation of cyclic nucleotide-mediated smooth muscle relaxation in Blacks as a cause of racial differences in vasodilator function. *Circulation, 99*, 90-95.

Carey, B.J., Eames, P.J., Blake, M.J., Panerai, R.B., & Potter, J.F. (2000). Dynamic cerebral autoregulation is unaffected by aging. *Stroke, 31*, 2895-2900.

Carlson, M.C., Fried, L.P., Xue, Q.L., Bandeen-Roche, K., Zeger, S.L., & Brandt, J. (1999). Association between executive attention and physical functional performance in community-dwelling older women. *Journal of Gerontology: Psychological Science & Social Science, 54*, S262-270.

Carro, E., Trejo, J.L., Busiguina, S., Torres-Aleman, I. (2001). Circulating insulin-like growth factor I mediates the protective effects of physical exercise against brain insults of different etiology and anatomy. *Journal of Neuroscience, 21(15)*, 5678-5684.

Carskadon, M.A., & Dement, W.C. (1992). Multiple sleep latency tests during the constant routine. *Sleep, 15(5)*, 396-399.

Casey, K.L. (1999). Forebrain mechanisms of nociception and pain: Analysis through imaging. *Proceedings of the National Academy of Sciences, 96(14)*, 7668-7674.

Caspersen, C.J. (1989). Physical activity epidemiology: Concepts, methods, and applications to exercise science. *Exercise & Sport Sciences Reviews, 18*, 439.

Caspersen, C.J., Merritt, R.K., & Stephens, T. (1994). International physical activity patterns: A methodological perspective. In R.K. Dishman (Ed.), *Advances in exercise adherence*. Champaign, IL: Human Kinetics.

Caspersen, C.J., Powell, K.E., Christenson, G.M. (1985). Physical activity, exercise, and physical fitness: Definitions and distinctions for health-related research. *Public Health Reports, 100*, 126-130.

References

Centers for Disease Control and Prevention. (2001). Physical activity trends: United States, 1990-1998. *Morbidity & Mortality Weekly Report, 50(09),* 166-169.

Cepeda, N.J., Kramer, A.F., & Gonzalez de Sather, J.C.M. (2001). Changes in executive control across the life span: Examination of task-switching performance. *Developmental Psychology, 37(5),* 715-730.

Cerella, J. (1990). Aging and information-processing rate. In J.E. Birren, & K.W. Schaie (Eds.), *Handbook of the psychology of aging* (3rd ed., pp. 201-221). San Diego, CA: Academic Press.

Cerella, J., Poon, L.W., & Williams, D. (1980). Age and the complexity hypothesis. In L.W. Poon (Ed.), *Aging in the 1980s: Psychological issues* (pp. 332-340). Washington, DC: American Psychological Assoc.

Cervilla, J.A., Prince, M., Joels, S., & Mann, A. (2000). Does depression predict cognitive outcome 9 to 12 years later? Evidence from a prospective study of elderly hypertensives. *Psychological Medicine, 30(5),* 1017-1023.

Chambliss, H.O., Van Hoomissen, J.D., Holmes, P.V., Bunnell, B.N., & Dishman, R.K. (2004). Effects of chronic activity wheel running and imipramine on male copulatory behavior after olfactory bulbectomy. *Physiology & Behavior, 82,* 593-600s.

Chance, B., Borer, E., Evans, A., Holtom, G., Kent, J., Maris, M., McCully, K., Northrop, J., & Shinkwin, M. (1989). Optical and nuclear magnetic resonance studies of hypoxia in human tissue and tumors. *Annals of the New York Academy of Sciences, 551,* 1-16.

Chaouloff, F., Laude, D., Serrurrier, B., Merino, D., Guezennec, C.Y., & Elghozi, J.L. (1987). Brain serotonin response to exercise in the rat: The influence of training duration. *Biogenic Amines, 4,* 99-106.

Chen, P., Ratcliff, G., Belle, S.H., Cauley, J.A., DeKosky, S.T., Ganguli, M. (2000). Cognitive tests that best discriminate between presymptomatic AD and those who remain nondemented. *Neurology, 55,* 1847-1853.

Chen, Y.C., Chen, Q.S., Lei, J.L., & Wang, S.L. (1998). Physical training modifies the age-related decrease of GAP-43 and synaptophysin in the hippocampal formation in C57BL/6J mouse. *Brain Research, 806,* 238-245.

Chennaoui, M., Drogou, C., Gomez-Merino, D., Gomez-Merino, D., Grimaldi, B., Fillion, G., & Guezennec, C.Y. (2001). Endurance training effects on 5-HT1B receptors mRNA expression in cerebellum, striatum, frontal cortex and hippocampus of rats. *Neuroscience Letters, 307(1),* 33-36.

Chennaoui, M., Grimaldi, B., Fillion, M.P., Bonnin, A., Drogou, C., Fillion, G., & Guezennec, C.Y. (2000). Effects of physical training on functional activity of 5-HT1b receptors in rat central nervous system. *Naunyn-Schmiedeberg's Archives of Pharmocology, 361,* 600-604.

Chodzko-Zajko, W.J. (1991). Physical fitness, cognitive performance and aging. *Medicine & Science in Sports & Exercise, 23,* 7.

Chodzko-Zajko, W.J. (2000). Successful aging in the new millennium: The role of regular physical activity. *Quest, 52,* 333-343.

Chodzko-Zajko, W.J., & Moore, K.A. (1994). Physical fitness and cognitive functioning in aging. *Exercise & Sport Sciences Reviews, 22,* 195-220.

References

Christensen, C., Frey, H.M., Foenstelien, E., Aadland, E., & Refsum, H.E. (1983). A critical evaluation of energy expenditure estimates based on individual O_2 consumption/heart rate curves and average daily heart rate. *American Journal of Clinical Nutrition, 37,* 468-472.

Clark, D.O. (1995). Racial and educational differences in physical activity among older adults. *Gerontologist, 35,* 472-480.

Clarkson-Smith, L., & Hartley, A.A. (1989). Relationships between physical exercise and cognitive abilities in older adults. *Psychology & Aging, 4,* 183-189.

Cohen, L.M. (1987). Diet and cancer. *Scientific American, 257,* 42-48.

Cohen-Zion, M., Stepnowsky, C., Marler, M., Shochat, T., Kripke, D.F., & Ancoli-Israel, S. (2001). Changes in cognitive function associated with sleep disordered breathing in older people. *Journal of the American Geriatrics Society, 49(12),* 1622-1627.

Colcombe, S.J., Erickson, K.I., Raz, N., Webb, A.G., Cohen, N.J., McAuley, E., & Kramer, A.F. (2003). Aerobic fitness reduces brain tissue loss in aging humans. *Journal of Gerontology: Biological Sciences & Medical Sciences, 58,* 176-180.

Colcombe, S.J., & Kramer, A.F. (2003). Fitness effects on the cognitive function of older adults: A meta-analytic study. *Psychological Science, 14,* 125-130.

Colier, W., Quaresima, V., Oeseburg, B., & Ferrari, M. (1999). Human motor-cortex oxygenation changes induced by cyclic coupled movements of the hand and foot. *Experimental Brain Research, 129,* 457-461.

Corwin, R.L., Robinson, J.K., & Crawley, J.N. (1993). Galanin antagonists block galanin-induced feeding in the hypothalamus and amygdala of the rat. *European Journal of Neuroscience, 5,* 1528-1533.

Cotman, C.W., & Berchtold, N.C. (2002). Exercise: A behavioral intervention to enhance brain health and plasticity. *Trends in Neurosciences, 25,* 295-301.

Cotman, C.W., & Engesser-Cesar, C. (2002). Exercise enhances and protects brain function. *Exercise & Sport Sciences Reviews, 30,* 75-79.

Craik, F.I.M. (1977). Age differences in human memory. In J.E. Birren & K.W. Schaie (Eds.), *Handbook of the psychology of aging* (pp. 384-420). New York: Van Nostrand Reinhold.

Craik, F.I.M., & Byrd, M. (1982). Aging and cognitive deficits: The role of attentional resources. In F.I.M. Craik & S. Trehub (Eds.), *Aging and cognitive processes.* New York: Plenum Press.

Craik, F.I.M., & Lockhart, R.S. (1972). Levels of processing: A framework for memory research. *Journal of Verbal Learning & Verbal Behavior, 11,* 671-684.

Crenshaw, M.C., & Edinger, J.D. (1999). Slow-wave sleep and waking cognitive performance among older adults with and without insomnia complaints. *Physiology & Behavior, 66(3),* 485-492.

Cress, M., Buchner, D., Questad, K., Esselman, P., de Lateur, B., & Schwartz, R. (1996). Continuous-scale physical functional performance in healthy older adults: A validation study. *Archives of Physical Medicine Rehabilitation, 77,* 1243-1250.

Cress, M.E., Buchner, D.M., Questad, K.A., Esselman, P.C., Schwartz, R.S., & de Lateur, B.J. (1999). Exercise: Effects on physical functional performance in independent older adults. *Journal of Gerontology: Medical Science, 54A(5),* M242-248.

References

Cress, M.E., & Meyer, M. (2003). Maximal voluntary and functional performance levels needed for independence in adults aged 65 to 97 years. *Journal of Physical Therapy, 83,* 37-48.

Cress, M.E., Schechtman, K.B., Mulrow, C.D., Fiatarone, M.A., Gerety, M.B., & Buchner, D.M. (1995). Relationship between physical performance and self-perceived physical function. *Journal of the American Geriatrics Society, 43,* 93-101.

Cricco, M., Simonsick, E.M., & Foley, D.J. (2001). The impact of insomnia on cognitive functioning in older adults. *Journal of the American Geriatrics Society, 49(9),* 1185-1189.

Critchley, H.D., Corfield, C.R., Chandler, M.P., Mathias, C.J., & Dolan, R.J. (2000). Cerebral correlates of autonomic cardiovascular arousal: A functional neuroimaging investigation in humans. *Journal of Physiology, 523,* 259-270.

Critchley, H.D., Melmed, R.N., Featherstone, E., Mathias, C.J., & Dolan, R.J. (2001). Brain activity during biofeedback relaxation: A functional neuroimaging investigation. *Brain, 124,* 1003-1012.

Crook, J., Rideout, E., & Browne, G. (1984). The prevalence of pain complaints in a general population. *Pain, 18(3),* 299-314.

Cruz-Casallas, P.E., Nasello, A.G., Hucke, E.E., & Felicio, L.F (1999). Dual modulation of male sexual behavior in rats by central prolactin: Relationship with in vivo striatal dopaminergic activity. *Psychoneuroendocrinology, 24(7),* 681-693.

Csernansky, J.G., Wang, L., Joshi, S., Miller, J.P., Gado, M., Kido, D., McKeel, D., Morris, J.C., & Miller, M.I. (2000). Early DAT is distinguished from ageing by high-dimensional mapping of the hippocampus. Dementia of the Alzheimer type. *Neurology, 55,* 1636-1643.

Davis, J.N., Carlsson, A., MacMillan, V., & Siesjo, B.K. (1973). Brain tryptophan hydroxylation: Dependence on arterial oxygen tension. *Science, 182,* 72-74.

Davis, J.N., Giron, L.T., Stanton, E., & Maury, W. (1979). The effect of hypoxia on brain neurotransmitter systems. In S. Fahn, J.N. Davis, & L.P. Rowland (Eds.), *Cerebral hypoxia and its consequences* (Vol. Advances in Neurology, 26, pp. 219-223). New York: Raven Press.

DeCastro, J.M., & Duncan, G. (1985). Operantly conditioned running: Effects on brain catecholamine concentrations and receptor densities in the rat. *Pharmacology, Biochemistry, & Behavior, 23,* 495-500.

deLeon, M.J., George, A.E., Ferris, S.H., Christman, D.R., Fowler, J.S., Gentes, C.I., Brodie, J., Reisberg, B., & Wolf, A.P. (1984). Positron emission tomography and computed tomography assessments of the aging human brain. *Journal of Computer Assisted Tomography, 8,* 88-94.

Dempster, F.N. (1992). The rise and fall of the inhibitory mechanism: Toward a unified theory of cognitive development and aging. *Developmental Review, 12,* 45-75.

Denio, L.S., Drake, M.E., & Pakalnis, A. (1989). The effect of exercise on seizure frequency. *Journal of Medicine, 20,* 171-176.

References

Derbyshire, S.W. (1999). Meta-analysis of thirty-four independent samples studied using PET reveals a significantly attenuated central response to noxious stimulation in clinical pain patients. *Current Review of Pain, 3(4),* 265-280.

Deutch, A.Y., & Bean, A.J. (1995). Colocalization in dopamine neurons. In F.E. Bloom & D.J. Kupfer (Eds.), *Psychopharmacology: The fourth generation of progress* (pp. 197-204). New York: Raven Press.

Deutsch, G., & Halsey, J.H. (1990). Cortical blood-flow effects of mental rotation in older subjects and Alzheimer patients. *Journal of Clinical and Experimental Neuropsychology, 12,* 31 [Abstract].

DeVito, G., Bernaradi, M., Forte, R., Pulejo, C, Macaluso, A, & Figura, F. (1998). Determinants of maximal instantaneous muscle power in women aged 50-75 years. *European Journal of Applied Physiology, 78(5),* 59-64.

DiGirolamo, G.J., Kramer, A.F., Barad, V., Cepeday, N.J., Weissman, D.H., Milham, M.P., Wszalek, T.M., Cohen, N.J., Banich, M.T., Webb, A., Belopolsky, A.V., & McAuley, E. (2001). General and task-specific frontal lobe recruitment in older adults during executive processes: A fMRI investigation of task-switching. *Neuroreport, 12,* 2065-2071.

Dinges, D.F., & Kribbs, N.B. (1991). Performing while sleepy: Effects of experimentally induced sleepiness. In Monk T.H. (Ed.), *Sleep, sleepiness and performance.* (pp. 97-128). New York: Wiley.

DiPietro, L. (2001). Physical activity in aging: Changes in patterns and their relationship to health and function. *Journal of Gerontology: Biological Sciences & Medical Sciences, 56 Spec No 2(2),* 13-22.

Dirnagl, U. (1997). Metabolic aspects of neurovascular coupling. In A. Villringer & U. Dirnagl (Eds.), *Optical imaging of brain function and metabolism* (Vol. II, pp. 155-159). New York: Plenum Press.

Dishman, R.K. (1994). The measurement conundrum in exercise adherence research. *Medicine & Science in Sports & Exercise, 26,* 1382-1390.

Dishman, R.K. (1997). Brain monoamines, exercise, and behavioral stress: Animal models. *Medicine & Science in Sports & Exercise, 29,* 63-74.

Dishman, R.K. (1997). The norepinephrine hypothesis. In W.P. Morgan (Ed.), *Physical activity and mental health* (pp. 199-212). Washington, DC: Taylor & Francis.

Dishman, R.K., Darracott, C.R., & Lambert, L.T. (1992). Failure to generalize determinants of self-reported physical activity to a motion sensor. *Medicine & Science in Sports & Exercise, 24,* 904-910.

Djousse, L., Ellison, R., McLennan, C., Cupples, L., Lipinska, I., Tofler, G., Gokce, N., & Vita, J. (1999). Acute effects of a high-fat meal with and without red wine on endothelial function in healthy subjects. *American Journal of Cardiology, 84,* 660-664.

Donohoe, R.T., & Benton, B. (2000). Glucose tolerance predicts performance on tests of memory and cognition. *Physiology & Behavior, 71,* 395-401.

Dorner, T., Brezinschek, H.P., Brezinschek, R.I., Foster, S.J., Domiati Saad, R., & Lipsky, P.E. (1997). Analysis of the frequency and pattern of somatic mutations within nonproductively rearranged human variable heavy chain genes. *Journal of Immunology, 158,* 2779-2789.

Drago, F., & Lissandrello, C.O. (2000). The "low-dose" concept and the paradoxical effects of prolactin on grooming and sexual behavior. *European Journal of Pharmacology, 405,* 131-137.

Duara, R., Barker, W.W., Chang, J., Yoshii, F., Loewenstein, D.A., & Pascal, S. (1992). Viability of neocortical function shown in behavioral activation state PET studies in Alzheimer disease. *Journal of Cerebral Blood Flow & Metabolism, 12,* 927-934.

Duara, R., Barker, W.W., Pascal, S., Loewenstein, D.A., & Boothe, T. (1990). Behavioral activation PET studies in normal aging and Alzheimer's disease. *Journal of Nuclear Medicine, 31,* 730.

Duman, R.S., Heninger, G.R., & Nestler, E.J. (1997). A molecular and cellular theory of depression. *Archives of General Psychiatry, 54,* 597-606.

Duman, R.S., & Nestler, E.J. (1995). Signal transduction pathways for catecholamine receptors. In F.E. Bloom, & D.J. Kupfer (Eds.), *Psychopharmacology: The fourth generation of progress* (pp. 303-320). New York: Raven Press.

Duncan, P.W., Weiner, D.K., Chandler, J., & Studenski, S. (1990). Functional reach: A new clinical measure of balance. *Journal of Gerontology: Medical Science, 45(6),* M192-M197.

Dustman, R.E., Emmerson, R.Y., Ruhling, R.O., Shearer, D.E., Steinhaus, L.A., Johnson, S.C., Bonekat, H.W., & Shigeoka, J.W. (1990). Age and fitness effects on EEG, ERPs, visual sensitivity, and cognition. *Neurobiology of Aging, 11,* 193-200.

Dustman, R.E., Emmerson, R.Y., & Shearer, D.E. (1990). Electrophysiology and aging: Slowing, inhibition, and aerobic fitness. In C.J. Brainerd (Ed.), *Cognitive and behavioral performance factors in atypical aging* (pp. 103-149). New York: Springer.

Dustman, R.E., Emmerson, R.Y., & Shearer, D.E. (1994). Physical activity, age and cognitive-neuropsychological function. *Journal of Aging & Physical Activity, 2,* 143-181.

Dustman, R.E., Emmerson, R.Y. and Shearer, D.E. (1996). Life span changes in electrophysiological measures of inhibition. *Brain & Cognition, 30,* 109-126.

Dustman, R.E., Ruhling, R.O., Russell, E.M., Shearer, D.E., Bonekat, H.W., Shigeoka, J.W., Wood, J.S., & Bradford, D.C. (1984). Aerobic exercise training and improved neuropsychological function of older individuals. *Neurobiology of Aging, 5,* 35-42.

Dustman, R.E., Shearer, D.E., & Emmerson, R.Y. (1993). EEG and event-related potentials in normal aging. *Progress in Neurobiology, 41,* 369-401.

Dustman, R.E., & Snyder, E.W. (1981). Life-span changes in visually evoked potentials at central scalp. *Neurobiology of Aging, 2,* 303-308.

Dustman, R.E., Snyder, E.W., & Schlehuber, C.J. (1981). Life-span alterations in visually evoked potentials and inhibitory function. *Neurobiology of Aging, 2,* 187-192.

Dutta, C., Hadley, E.C., & Lexell, J. (1997). Sarcopenia and physical performance in old age: Overview. *Muscle & Nerve, 5,* S5-S9.

Dwyer, J. (1995). Genes, blood pressure, and African heritage. *Lancet, 346,* 392.

Dwyer, D., & Browning, J. (2000). Endurance training in Wistar rats decreases receptor sensitivity to a serotonin agonist. *Acta Physiologica Scandanavica, 170(3),* 211-216

Dywan, J., & Murphy, W.E. (1996). Aging and inhibitory control in text comprehension. *Psychology & Aging, 11,* 199-206.

Eaton, S.B., Konner, M., & Shostak, M. (1988). Stone Agers in the fast lane: Chronic degenerative diseases in evolutionary perspective. *American Journal of Medicine, 84,* 739-749.

Eccleston, C. (1995). Chronic pain and distraction: An experimental investigation into the role of sustained and shifting attention in the processing of chronic persistent pain. *Behavioral Research & Therapy, 33(4),* 391-405.

Eccleston, C., & Crombez, G. (1999). Pain demands attention: A cognitive-affective model of the interruptive function of pain. *Psychological Bulletin, 125(3),* 356-366.

Edinger, J.D., Morey, M.C., Sullivan, R.J., Higginbotham, M.B., Marsh, G.R., Dailey, D.S., & McCall, W.V. (1993). Aerobic fitness, acute exercise and sleep in older men. *Sleep, 16(4),* 351-359.

Ellermann, J., Garwood, M., Hendrich, K., Hinke, R., Hu, X., King, S.G., Menon, R., Merkle, H., Ogawa, S., & Ugurbil, K. (1994). Functional imaging of the brain by nuclear magnetic resonance. In R. Gillies (Ed.), *NMR in physiology and biomedicine* (pp. 137-150). San Diego: Academic Press.

Emery, C.F., (1994). Effects of age on physiological and psychological functioning among COPD patients in an exercise program. *Journal of Aging & Health, 6,* 3-16.

Emery, C.F., & Blumenthal, J.A. (1990). Perceived change among participants in an exercise program for older adults. *Gerontologist, 30(4),* 516-521.

Emery, C.F., Burker, E.J., & Blumenthal, J.A. (1991). Psychological and physiological effects of exercise among older adults. In K.W. Schaie (Ed.), *Annual review of gerontology and geriatrics,* 11 (pp. 218-238). New York: Springer.

Emery, C.F., Leatherman, N.E., Burker, E.J., & MacIntyre, N.R. (1991). Psychological outcomes of a pulmonary rehabilitation program. *Chest, 100(3),* 613-617.

Emery, C.F., Schein, R.L., Hauck, E.R., & MacIntyre, N.R. (1998). Psychological and cognitive outcomes of a randomized trial of exercise among patients with chronic obstructive pulmonary disease. *Health Psychology, 17(3),* 232-240.

Ergul, A., Shoemaker, K., Puett, D., & Tackett, R. (1998). Gender differences in the expression of endothelin receptors in human saphenous veins in vitro. *Journal of Pharmacology & Experimental Therapeutics, 285(2),* 511-517.

Ergul, A., Tackett, R., & Puett, D. (1999). Distribution of endothelin receptors in saphenous veins of African Americans: Implications of racial differences. *Journal of Cardiovascular Pharmacology, 34,* 327-332.

Eriksen, H.R., Ellertsen, B., Grønningsaeter, H., Nakken, K.O., Løyning, Y., & Ursin, H. (1994). Physical exercise in women with intractable epilepsy. *Epilepsia, 35,* 1256-1264.

References

Ernest, J.T., & Krill, A.E. (1971). The effect of hypoxia on visual function. *Investigative Ophthalmology, 10,* 323-328.

Etnier, J.L., & Berry M. (2001). Fluid intelligence in an older COPD sample after short- or long-term exercise. *Medicine & Science in Sports & Exercise, 33(10),* 1620-1628.

Etnier, J.L., Salazar, W., Landers, D.M., Petruzzello, S.J., Han, M., & Nowell, P. (1997). The influence of physical fitness and exercise upon cognitive functioning: A meta-analysis. *Journal of Sport & Exercise Psychology, 19,* 249-277.

Ettinger, W.H., Burns, R., Messier, S.P., Applegate, W., Rejeski, W.J., Morgan, T., Shumaker, S., Berry, M.J., O'Toole, M., Monu, J., & Craven, T. (1997). A randomized trial comparing aerobic exercise and resistance exercise with a health education program in older adults with knee osteoarthritis. *Journal of the American Medical Association, 277(1),* 25-31.

Farmer, M.E., Locke, B.Z., Moscicki, E.K., Dannenberg, A.L., Larson, D.B., & Radloff, L.S. (1988). Physical activity and depressive symptoms: The NHANES I epidemiologic follow-up study. *American Journal of Epidemiology, 128(6),* 1340-1351.

Fazeka, F., Alavi, A., Chawluk, J.B., Zimmerman, R.A., Hackney, D., Bilaniuk, L., Rosen, M., Alves, W.M., Hurtig, H.I., Jamieson, D.G., Kushner, M.J., & Reivich, M. (1989). Comparison of CT, MR, and PET in Alzheimer dementia and normal aging. *Journal of Nuclear Medicine, 30,* 1607-1615.

Femia, E.E., Zarit, S.H., & Johansson, B. (2001). The disablement process in very late life: A study of the oldest-old in Sweden. *Journal of Gerontology: Psychological Sciences, 56B(1),* P12-P23.

Ferris, S.H., deLeon, M.J., Wolf, A.P., George, A.E., Reisberg, B., Christman, D.R., Yonekura, Y. & Fowler, S. (1983). Positron emission tomography in dementia. *Advances in Neurology, 38,* 123-129.

Fiatarone, M.A., O'Neill, E.F., Ryan, N.D., Clements, K.M., Solares, G. R., Nelson, M.E., Roberts, S.B., Kehayias, J.J., Lipsitz, L.A., & Evans, W. J. (1994). Exercise training and nutritional supplementation for physical frailty in very elderly people. *New England Journal of Medicine, 330,* 1769-1775.

Fix, A.J., Golden, C.J., Daughton, D., Kass, I., & Bell, C.W. (1982). Neuropsychological deficits among patients with chronic obstructive pulmonary disease. *International Journal of Neuroscience, 16(2),* 99-105.

Fletcher, R.C. (2000). *The functional neuroimaging of memory disorder.* In J.C., Mazziotta, A.W. Toga, & R.S.J. Frackowiak, (Eds.), *Brain mapping: The disorders* (pp 201-215). San Diego,CA: Academic Press.

Foldvari, M., Clark, M., Laviolette, L.C., Bernstein, M.A., Kaliton, D., Castaneda, C., Pu, C.T., Hausdorff, J.M., Fielding, R.A., & Sing, M.A. (2000). Association of muscle power with functional status in community-dwelling elderly women. *Journal of Gerontology: Medical Sciences, 55A(4),* M192-M199.

Folkins, C.H., & Sime, W.E. (1981). Physical fitness training and mental health. *American Psychologist, 36,* 373-389.

Foote, S.L., & Aston-Jones, G.S. (1995). Pharmacology and physiology of central noradrenergic systems. In F.E. Bloom & D.J. Kupfer (Eds.), *Psychopharmacology: The fourth generation of progress* (pp. 335-345). New York: Raven Press.

Fordyce, D.E., & Farrar, R.P. (1991). Physical activity effects on hippocampal and parietal cortical cholinergic function and spatial learning in F344 rats. *Behavioural Brain Research, 43,* 115-123.

Fordyce, D.E., Starnes, J.W., & Farrar R.P. (1991). Compensation of the age-related decline in hippocampal mascarinic receptor density through daily exercise or underfeeding. *Journal of Gerontology: Psychological Science & Social Science, 46,* B245-248.

Fordyce, D.E., & Wehner, J.M. (1993). Physical activity enhances spatial learning performance with an associated alteration in hippocampal protein kinase C activity in C57BL/6 and DBA/2 mice. *Brain Research, 619,* 111-119.

Foster, N.L., Chase, T.N., Fedio, P., Patronas, N.J., Brooks, R.A., & Di Chiro, G. (1983). Alzheimer's disease: Focal cortical changes shown by positron emission tomography. *Neurology 33,* 961-965.

Frackowiak, R.S.J., Lenzi, G.L., Jones, T., & Heather, J.D. (1980). Quantitative measurement of regional cerebral blood flow and oxygen metabolism in man using ^{15}O and positron emission tomography: Theory, procedure, and normal values. *Journal of Computer Assisted Tomography, 4,* 727-736.

Freedson, P.S., & Miller, K. (2000). Objective monitoring of physical activity using motion sensors and heart rate. *Research Quarterly for Exercise & Sport, 71,* 21-29.

Fried, L.P., Herdman, S.J., Kuhn, K.E., Rubin, G., & Turano, K. (1991). Preclinical disability: Hypotheses about the bottom of the iceberg. *Journal of Aging & Health, 3(2),* 285-300.

Friedland, R.P. (1990). Brain imaging and cerebral metabolism. In F. Boller, & J. Grafman (Eds.), *Handbook of neuropsychology* (pp. 197-211). North Holland, Amsterdam: Elsevier Science.

Frier, B.M. (2001). Hypoglycaemia and cognitive function in diabetes. *International Journal of Clinical Practice, 123(Suppl.),* 30-37.

Gallo, J.J., & Lebowitz, B.D. (1999). The epidemiology of common late-life mental disorders in the community: Themes for the new century. *Psychiatric Services, 50(9),* 1158-1166.

Garfinkel, M.S., Singhal, A., Katz, W.A., Allan, D.A., Reshetar, R., & Schumacher, H.R. (1998). Yoga-based intervention for carpal tunnel syndrome: A randomized trial. *Journal of the American Medical Association, 280(18),* 1601-1603.

Gauchard, G.C., Jeandel, C., Tessier, A., & Perrin, P.P. (1999). Beneficial effect of proprioceptive physical activities on balance control in elderly human subjects. *Neuroscience Letters, 273(2),* 81-84.

Gayle, R., Montoye, H.J., & Philpot, J. (1977). Accuracy of pedometers for measuring distance walked. *American Alliance for Health, Physical Education, & Recreation Research Quarterly, 48,* 632-636.

Gerety, M.B., Mulrow, C.D., Ruley, M.R., Hazuda, H.P., Lichtenstein, M.J., & Bohannon, R. (1993). Development and validation of a physical performance instrument for the functionally impaired elderly: The Physical Disability Index (PDI). *Journal of Gerontology: Medical Sciences, 48(2),* M33-M38.

References

Giacca, A., Shi, Z.Q., Marliss, E.B., Zinman, B., & Vranic, M. (1994). Physical activity, fitness, and Type I Diabetes. In C. Bouchard, R.J. Shephard, & T. Stephens (Eds.), *Physical, activity, fitness and health: International proceedings and consensus statement* (pp. 656-668). Champaign, IL: Human Kinetics.

Gibson, G.E., & Peterson, C. (1982). Biochemical and behavioral parallels in aging and hypoxia. In E. Giacobini, G. Filogamo, G. Giacobini, & A. Vernadakis (Eds.), *Cellular and molecular mechanisms of aging in the nervous system* (pp. 107-122). New York: Raven Press.

Gill, T.M., Richardson, E.D., & Tinetti, ME. (1995). Evaluating the risk of dependence in activities of daily living among community-living older adults with mild to moderate cognitive impairment. *Journal of Gerontology: Medical Sciences, 50A(5)*, M235-M241.

Gill, T.M., Williams, C.S., Richardson, E.D., & Tinetti, ME. (1996). Impairments in physical performance and cognitive status as predisposing factors for functional dependence among nondisabled older persons. *Journal of Gerontology: Medical Sciences, 51A(6)*, M283-M288.

Gilliam, P.E., Spirduso, W.W., Martin, T.P., Walters, T.J., Wilcox, R.E., & Farrar, R.P. (1984). The effects of exercise training on [^{3}H]-spiperone binding in rat striatum. *Pharmacology, Biochemistry, & Behavior, 20*, 863-867.

Glaser, G.H. (1963). The normal electroencephalogram and its reactivity. In G.H. Glaser (Ed.), *EEG and behavior* (pp. 3-23). New York: Basic Books.

Globus, M., Melamed, E., Keren, A., Tzivone, D., Granot, C., Lavy, S., et al. (1983). Effect of exercise on cerebral circulation. *Journal of Cerebral Blood Flow & Metabolism, 3*, 287-290.

Göetze, W., Kubicki, S., Munter, M., & Teichmann, J. (1967). Effect of physical exercise on seizure threshold. *Epilepsia, 28*, 664-667.

Gold, P.E. (1995). Role of glucose in regulating the brain and cognition. *American Journal of Clinical Nutrition, 61(Suppl.)*, 987S-995S.

Goldberg, A.P., & Hagberg, J.M. (1990). Physical exercise and the elderly. In E.L. Schneider, & J.W. Rowe (Eds.), *Handbook of the biology of aging* (pp. 407-423). San Diego: Academic Press,

Goldstein, G., & Shelly, C.H. (1975). Similarities and differences between psychological deficit in aging and brain damage. *Journal of Gerontology, 30*, 448-455.

Golomb, J., Kluger, A., deLeon, M.J., Ferris, S., Convit, A., Mittelman, M., Cohen, J., Rusinek, H., de Santi, S., & George, A. (1994). Hippocampal formation size in normal human aging: A correlate of delayed secondary memory performance. *Learning & Memory, 1*, 45-54.

Good, C.D., Johnsrude, I.S., Ashburner, J., Henson, R.N., Friston, K.J., & Frackowiak, R.S.J. (2001). A voxel-based morphometric study of ageing in 465 normal adult human brains. *Neuroimage, 14*, 21-36.

Gopalan, C., Tian, Y., Moore, K.E., & Lookingland, K.J. (1993). Neurochemical evidence that the inhibitory effect of galanin on tuberinfundibular dopamine is activity-dependent. *Neuroendocrinology, 58(3)*, 287-293.

Grady, C.L., Haxby, J., Horwitz, B., Gillette, J., Salerno, J., Gonzalez-Aviles, A., Carson, R., Herscovitch, P., Schapiro, M., & Rapoport, S. (1993). Activation of cerebral blood flow during a visuoperceptual task in patients with Alzheimer-type dementia. *Neurobiology of Aging, 14,* 35-44.

Grady, C.L., Maisog, J., Horwitz, B., Ungerleider, L., Mentis, M.J., Salerno, J.A., Pietrini, P., Wagner, H.N., Jr., & Haxby, J.V. (1994). Age-related changes in cortical blood flow activation during visual processing of faces and location. *Journal of Neuroscience, 14,* 1450-1462.

Grady, C.L., McIntosh, A.R., Bookstein, F., Horwitz, B., Rapoport, S., & Haxby, J.V. (1998). Age-related changes in regional cerebral blood flow during working memory for faces. *Neuroimage, 8,* 409-425.

Grady, C.L., McIntosh, A.R., Horwitz, B., Maisog, J.M., Ungerleider, L.G., Mentis, M.J., Pietrini, P., Schapiro, M.B., & Haxby, J.V. (1995). Age-related reductions in human recognition memory due to impaired encoding. *Science, 269,* 218-221.

Grady, C.L., McIntosh, A.R., Horwitz, B., & Rapoport, S. I. (2000). Age-related changes in the neural correlates of degraded and non-degraded face processing. *Cognitive Neuropsychology, 217,* 165-186.

Grassi, B.M., Quaresima, V., Marconi, C., Ferrari, M., & Cerretelli, P. (1999). Blood lactate accumulation and muscle deoxygenation during incremental exercise. *Journal of Applied Physiology, 87,* 348-355.

Gretebeck, R.J., & Montoye, H.J., & Porter, W. (1991). Comparison of doubly labeled Water method for measuring energy expenditure with Caloric accelerometer recordings [Abstract]. *Medicine & Science in Sports & Exercise, 23,* S60.

Grossman, M., Cooke, A., DeVita, C, Alsop, D., Detre, J., Chen, W., & Gee, J. (2002). Age-related changes in working memory during sentence comprehension: An fMRI study. *Neuroimage, 15,* 302-317.

Gundlach, A.L., & Burazin, T.C. (1998). Galanin-galanin receptor systems in the hypothalamic paraventricular and supraoptic nuclei: Some recent findings and future challenges. *Annals of the New York Academy of Sciences, 863,* 241-251.

Guralnik, J.M., & Simonsick, E.M. (1993). Physical disability in older Americans. *Journal of Gerontology: Medical Sciences, 48,* 3-10.

Guralnik, J.M., Simonsick, E.M., Ferrucci, L., Glynn, R.J., Berkman, L. F., Blazer, D.G., Scherr, P.A., & Wallace, R.B. (1994). A short physical performance battery assessing lower extremity function: Association with self-reported disability and prediction of mortality and nursing home admission. *Journal of Gerontology: Medical Sciences, 49(2),* M85-M94.

Gutin, B. (1972). Exercise-induced activation and human performance: A review. *Research Quarterly, 44,* 256-268.

Guttmann, C.R.G., Jolesz, F.A., Kikinis, R., Killiany, R.J., Moss, M.B., Sandor, T., & Albert, M.S. (1998). White matter changes with normal aging. *Neurology, 50,* 972-978.

Haan, M.N., & Weldon, M. (1996). The influence of diabetes, hypertension, and stroke on ethnic differences in physical and cognitive functioning in an ethnically diverse older population. *Annals of Epidemiology, 6(5),* 392-398.

Hale, S., Myerson, J., & Wagstaff, D. (1987). General slowing of nonverbal information processing: Evidence for a power law. *Journal of Gerontology, 42,* 131-136.

Hall, C.D., Smith, A.L., & Keele, S.W. (2001). The impact of aerobic activity on cognitive function in older adults: A new synthesis based on the concept of executive control. *European Journal of Cognitive Psychology, 13*, 279-300.

Hall, J.L., & Gold, P.E. (1986). The effects of training, epinephrine, and glucose injections on plasma glucose levels in rats. *Behavioral & Neural Biology, 46*, 156-157.

Hall, J.L., Gonder-Frederick, L.A., Chewning, W.W., Silveira, J., & Gold, P.E. (1989). Glucose enhancement of performance on memory tests in young and aged humans. *Neuropsychologia, 27*, 1129-1138.

Haller, J.W., Christensen, G.E., Joshi, S.C., et al. (1996). Hippocampal MR imaging morphometry by means of general pattern matching. *Radiology, 199*, 787-791.

Harms, M., Colier, W., Wieling, W., Lenders, J., Scecher, N., & van Lieshout, J. (2000). Orthostatic tolerance, cerebral oxygenation, and blood velocity in humans with sympathetic failure. *Stroke, 31*, 1608-1614.

Harnishfeger, K.K., & Pope, R.S. (1996). Intending to forget: The development of cognitive inhibition in directed forgetting. *Journal of Experimental Child Psychology, 62*, 292-315.

Hart, R.P., Martelli, M.F., & Zasler, N.D. (2000). Chronic pain and neuropsychological functioning. *Neuropsychology Review, 10(3)*, 131-149.

Hasher, L., & Zacks, R.T. (1979). Automatic and effortful processes in memory. *Journal of Experimental Psychology: General, 108*, 350-388.

Hasher, L., & Zacks, R.T. (1988). Working memory, comprehension, and aging: A review and a new view. In G.H. Bower (Ed.), *The psychology of learning and motivation* (Vol. 22, pp. 193-226). San Diego: Academic Press.

Haskell, W.L., Yee, M.C., Evans, A., & Irby, P.J. (1993). Simultaneous measurement of heart rate and body motion to quantitate physical activity. *Medicine & Science in Sports & Exercise, 25*, 109-115.

Hausdorff, J.J., Nelson, M.E., Kaliton, D., Layne, J.E., Berstein, M.J., Nuernberger, A., & Fiatarone Singh, M.A. (2001). Etiology and modification of gait instability in older adults: A randomized trial of exercise. *Journal Applied Physiology, 90*, 2117-2129.

Hawkins, H., Kramer, A.F., & Capaldi, D. (1992). Aging, exercise, and attention. *Psychology & Aging, 7*, 643-653.

Haynie, D.A., Berg, S., Johansson, B., Gatz, M., & Zarit, S.H. (2001). Symptoms of depression in the oldest old: A longitudinal study. *Journal of Gerontology: Psychological Science & Social Science, 56(2)*, P111-1118.

Heimer, L., Zahm, D., & Alheid, G. (1995). Basal ganglia. In G. Paxinos (Ed.), *The rat nervous system* (2nd ed., pp. 579-628). Sidney: Academic Press

Helme, R.D., & Gibson, S.J. (1999). *Pain in older people*. In I.K. Crombie (Ed.), *Epidemiology of Pain* (pp. 103-112). Seattle: IASP Press.

Hendelman, D., Miller, K., Baggett, C., Debold, E., & Freedson, P. (2000). Validity of accelerometry for the assessment of moderate intensity physical activity in the field. *Medicine & Science in Sports & Exercise, 32, (Suppl.)*, S442-S449.

Hertzog, C., & Bleckley, M.K. (2001). Age differences in the structure of intelligence: Influences of information processing speed. *Intelligence, 29*, 191-217.

References

Heyer, E.J., Sharma, R., Winfree, C.J., Mocco, J., McMahon, D.J., McCormick, P.A., Quest, D.O., McMurtry, J.G. 3rd, Riedel, C.J., Lazar, R.M., Stern, Y., & Connolly, E.S., Jr. (2000). Severe pain confounds neuropsychological test performance. *Journal of Clinical & Experimental Neuropsychology, 22(5)*, 633-639.

Hoffmann, P. (1997). The endorphin hypothesis. In W.P. Morgan (Ed.), *Physical activity and mental health* (pp. 163-176). Washington, DC: Taylor & Francis.

Hokfelt, T., Broberger, C., Xu, Z.D., Sergeyev, V., Ubink, R., & Diez, M. (2000). Neuropeptides: An overview. *Neuropharmacolology, 39*, 1337-1356.

Holets, V.R., Hokfelt, T., Rokaeus, A., Terenius, L., & Goldstein, M. (1988). Locus coeruleus neurons in the rat containing neuropeptide Y, tyrosine hydroxylase or galanin and their efferent projections to the spinal cord, cerebral cortex and hypothalamus. *Neuroscience, 24*, 893-906.

Holmes, P.V., & Crawley, J.N. (1995). Coexisting neurotransmitters in central noradrenergic neurons. In F.E. Bloom, & D.J. Kupfer (Eds.), *Psychopharmacology: The fourth generation of progress* (pp. 347-353). New York: Raven Press.

Horn, J.L., & Cattell, R.B. (1972). Age differences in fluid and crystallized intelligence. *Acta Psychologica Scandanavica, 26*, 103-129.

Horvitz, M.A., & Schoeller, D.A. (2001). Natural abundance deuterium and 18-oxygen effects on the precision of the doubly labeled water method. *American Journal of Physiology, Endocrinology, & Metabolism, 280*, E965-E972.

Houtman, S., Colier, W., Hopman, M., & Oeseburg, B. (1999). Reproducibility of the alterations in circulation and cerebral oxygenation from supine rest to head-up tilt. *Clinical Physiology, 19*, 169-177.

Houtman, S., Serrador, J.M., Colier, W.N., Strijbos, D.W., Shoemaker, K., & Hopman, M.T. (2001). Changes in cerebral oxygenation and blood flow during LBNP in spinal cord-injured individuals. *Journal of Applied Physiology, 91*, 2199-2205.

Hubel, D.H. (1988). *Eye, Brain, and Vision* (Vol. 22). New York: Scientific American Library.

Hubel, D.H., & Wiesel, T.N. (1962). Receptive fields, binocular interaction and functional architecture in the cat's visual cortex. *Journal of Physiology, 106*, 106-154.

Humphries, A., deWolfe, V., Young, J., & LeFevre, F. (1963). Evaluation of the natural history and the results of treatment in occlusive arteriosclerosis involving the lower extremities in 1,850 patients. In S. Wesolowski, & C. Dennis (Eds.), *Fundamentals of vascular grafting.* (pp. 423-440). New York: McGraw-Hill.

Ide, K., Horn, A., & Secher, N.H. (1998). Cerebral metabolic response to sub-maximal exercise. *Journal of Applied Physiology, 87*, 1604-1608.

Ide, K., & Secher, N.H. (2000). Cerebral blood flow and metabolism during exercise. *Progress in Neurobiology, 61*, 397-414.

Ingram, D. (1988). Key questions in developing biomarkers of aging. *Experimental Gerontology, 23*, 429-434.

Itoh, M., Hatazawa, J., Miyazawa, H., Matsui, H., Meguro, K., Yanai, K., et al. (1990). Stability of cerebral blood flow and oxygen metabolism during normal aging. *Gerontology, 36*, 43-48.

References

Jacobs, B.L., & Fornal, C.A. (1995). Serotonin and behavior a general hypothesis. In F.E. Bloom & D.J. Kupfer (Eds.), *Psychopharmacology: The fourth generation of progress* (pp. 461-469). New York: Raven Press.

Jacobs, D.R., Ainsworth, B.E., Hartman, T.J., & Leon, A.S. (1993). A simultaneous evaluation of 10 commonly used physical activity questionnaires. *Medicine & Science in Sports & Exercise, 25*, 81-91.

Jamieson, D.G., Chawluk, J.B., Alavi, A., Hurtig, H.I., Rosen, M., Bais, S. Dann, R., Kushner, M., & Reivich, M. (1987). The effect of disease severity on local cerebral glucose metabolism in Alzheimer disease. *Journal of Cerebral Blood Flow & Metabolism, 7(Suppl. 1)*, S410.

Jang, Y., Mortimer, J.A., Haley, W.E., Chisolm, T.E.H., & Graves, A.B. (2002). Nonauditory determinants of self-perceived hearing problems among older adults: The role of stressful life conditions, neuroticism, and social resources. *Journal of Gerontology: Medical Sciences, 57A(7)*, M466-M469.

Jelicic, M., Bosma, H., Ponds, R.W., Van Boxtel, M.P., Houx, P.J., & Jolles, J. (2002). Subjective sleep problems in later life as predictors of cognitive decline. Report from the Maastricht Ageing Study (MAAS). *International Journal of Geriatric Psychiatry, 7(1)*, 73-77.

Jernigan, T.L., Archibald, S.L. Fennema-Notesting, C., Gamst, A.C., Stout, J.C., Bonner, J., & Hesselink, J.R. (2001). Effects of age on tissues and regions of the cerebrum and cerebellum. *Neurobiology of Aging, 22*, 581-594.

Jette, A.M., Jette, D.U., Ng, J., Plotkin, D.J., & Bach, M.A. (1999). Are performance-based measures sufficiently reliable for use in multicenter trials? *Journal of Gerontology: Medical Sciences, 54A(1)*, M3-M6.

Jette, A.M., Lachman, M., Giorgetti, M.M., Assmann, S.F., Harris, B.A., Levenson, C., Wernick, M., & Krebs, D. (1999). Exercise: It's never too late. The strong-for-life program. *American Journal Public Health, 89(1)*, 66-72.

Jiang, A.-L., Yamaguchi, H., Tanaka, H., Takahashi, A., Tanabe, S., Utsuyama, N., et al. (1995). Blood flow velocity in the common carotid artery in humans during graded exercise on a treadmill. *European Journal of Applied Physiology, 70*, 234-239.

Johanson, D.C., & Edey, M.A. (1981). *Lucy, the beginnings of humankind.* New York: Simon & Schuster.

Johnson, S.C., Saykin, A.J., Baxter, L.C., Flashman, L.A., Santulli, R.B., McAllister, T.W., & Mamourian, AC. (2000). The relationship between fMRI activation and cerebral atrophy: Comparison of normal aging and Alzheimer disease. *NeuroImage, 11*, 179-187.

Johnston, A.N.B., & Rose, S.P.R. (2001). Memory consolidation in day-old chicks requires BDNF but not NGF or NT-3: An antisense study. *Molecular Brain Research, 88*, 26-36.

Jonsdottir, I.H. (2000). Neuropeptides and their interaction with exercise and immune function. *Immunology & Cell Biology, 78*, 562-570.

Jorgensen, L.G., Perko, G., & Secher, N.H. (1992). Regional cerebral artery mean flow velocity and blood flow during dynamic exercise in humans. *Journal of Applied Physiology, 73*, 1825-1830.

References

Kanarek, R.B., Gerstein, A.V., Wildman, R.P., Mathes, W.F., & D'Anci, K.E. (1998). Chronic running-wheel activity decreases sensitivity to morphine-induced analgesia in male and female rats. *Pharmacology, Biochemistry, & Behavior, 61,* 19-27.

Kaplan, G.A. (1997). *Behavioral, social, and environmental factors adding years to life and life to years.* Baltimore, MD: Johns Hopkins Press.

Karacan, I., Thornby, J.I., Anch, M., Holzer, C.E., Warheit, G.J., Schwab, J.J., & Williams, R.L. (1976). Prevalence of sleep disturbance in a primarily urban Florida County. *Social Science & Medicine, 10(5),* 239-244.

Kennedy, D.O., & Scholey, A.B. (2000). Glucose administration, heart rate and cognitive performance: Effects of increasing mental effort. *Psychopharmacology, 149,* 63-71.

Kenney, L., & Ho, C.W. (1995). Age alters regional distribution of blood flow during moderate-intensity exercise. *Journal of Applied Physiology, 79,* 1112-1119.

Kessler, J., Herholz, K., Grond, M., & Heiss, W.D. (1991). Impaired metabolic-activation in Alzheimer's Disease—A PET study during continuous visual recognition. *Neuropsychologia, 29,* 229-243.

Kessler, R.C., McGonagle, K.A., Zhao, S., Nelson, C.B., Hughes, M., Eshleman, S., Wittchen, H.U., & Kendler, K.S. (1994). Lifetime and 12-month prevalence of DSM-III-R psychiatric disorders in the United States. Results from the National Comorbidity Survey. *Archives of General Psychiatry, 51(1),* 8-19.

Keysor, J.J., & Jette, A.M. (2001). Have we oversold the benefit of late-life exercise? *Journal of Gerontology: Medical Sciences, 56A(7),* M412-M423.

King, A.C., Baumann, K., O'Sullivan, P., Wilcox, S., & Castro, C. (2002). Effects of moderate-intensity exercise on physiological, behavioral, and emotional responses to family caregiving: A randomized controlled trial. *Journal of Gerontology: Biological Science Medical Science, 57A(1),* M26-36.

King, A.C., Oman, R.F., Brassington, G.S., Bliwise, D.L., & Haskell, W.L. (1997). Moderate-intensity exercise and self-rated quality of sleep in older adults. A randomized controlled trial. *Journal of the American Medical Association, 277(1),* 32-37.

King, D.A., Cox, C., Lyness, J.M., & Caine, E.D. (1995). Neuropsychological effects of depression and age in an elderly sample: A confirmatory study. *Neuropsychology, 9,* 339-408.

Kleinschmidt, A., Obrig, H., Requardt, M., Merboldt, K.D., Dirnagl, U., Villringer, A., & Frahm, J. (1996). Simultaneous recording of cerebral blood oxygenation changes during human brain activation by magnetic resonance imaging and near-infrared spectroscopy. *Journal of Cerebral Blood Flow & Metabolism, 16,* 817-826.

Koenig, H.G., & Blazer, D.G. (1992). Epidemiology of geriatric affective disorders. *Clinical Geriatric Medicine, 8(2),* 235-251.

Kollokian, V. (1996). Performance analysis of automatic techniques for tissue classification in magnetic resonance images of the human brain. Department of Computer Science, Concordia University, Montreal, Quebec, Canada. As cited in Mega, M.S., Thompson, P.M., Toga, A.W., & Cummings, J.L. (2000). *Brain mapping in dementia.* In A.W. Toga, & J.C. Mazziotta (Eds.), *Brain mapping: The systems.* (pp. 217-239). San Diego, CA: Academic Press.

References

Koltyn, K.F. (1997). The thermogenic hypothesis. In W.P. Morgan (Ed.), *Physical activity and mental health* (pp. 213-226). Washington, DC: Taylor & Francis.

Koltyn, K.F. (2002). Using physical activity to manage pain in older adults. *Journal of Aging & Physical Activity, 10,* 226-239.

Kramer, A.F., Colcombe, S., Erickson, K., Belopolsky, A., McAuley, E., Cohen, N.J., Webb, A., Jerome, G.J., Marquez, D.X., & Wszalek, T.M. (2002). Effects of aerobic fitness training on human cortical function: A proposal. *Journal of Molecular Neuroscience, 19,* 227-231.

Kramer, A.F., Hahn, S., Cohen, N.J., Banich, M.T., McAuley, E., Harrison, C.R., et al. (1999). Aging, fitness and neurocognitive function. *Nature, 400,* 418-419.

Kramer, A.F., Hahn, S., & Gopher, D. (1999). Task coordination and aging: Explorations of executive control processes in the task switching paradigm. *Acta Psychologica, 101,* 339-378.

Kramer, A.F., Hahn, S., & McAuley, E. (2000). Influence of aerobic fitness on the neurocognitive function of older adults. *Journal of Aging & Physical Activity, 8 (4),* 379-385.

Kramer, A.F., Hahn, S., McAuley, E., Cohen, N. J., Banich, M.T., Harrison, C., et al. (2002). Exercise, aging, and cognition: Healthy body, healthy mind? In W.A. Rogers & A.D. Fisk (Eds.), *Human factors interventions for health care of older adults.* (pp. 91-120). Mahwah, NJ: Lawrence Erlbaum.

Kramer, A.F., Sowon, H., Cohen, N.J., Banich, M.T., McAuley, E., Harrison, C.R., Chason, J., Vakil, E., Bardell, L., Boileau, R.A., & Colcombe, A. (1999). Ageing, fitness, and neurocognitive function. *Nature, 400,* 418-419.

Kramer, A.F., & Willis, S.L. (2002). Enhancing the cognitive vitality of older adults. *Current Directions in Psychological Science, 11,* 173-176.

Kramer, J.M., Beatty, J.A., Plowey, E.D., & Waldrop, T.G. (2002). Exercise and hypertension: A model for central neural plasticity. *Clinical & Experimental Pharmacology & Physiology, 29,* 122-126.

Kremkau, F. (1998). *Diagnostic ultrasound: Principles and practice* (5th ed.). Philadelphia: W.B. Saunders.

Kutner, N.G., Barnhart, H., Wolf, S.L., McNeely, E., & Xu, T. (1997). Self-report benefits of Tai Chi practice by older adults. *Journal of Gerontology: Psychological Sciences, 52(5),* 242-246.

Landers, D.M., & Petruzzello, S.J. (1994). Physical activity, fitness, and anxiety. In C. Bouchard, R.J. Shephard, & T. Stephens (Eds.), *Physical, activity, fitness and health: International proceedings and consensus statement* (pp. 868-882). Champaign, IL: Human Kinetics.

LaPorte, R.E., Montoye, H.J., & Caspersen, C.J. (1985). Assessment of physical activity in epidemiologic research: Problems and prospects. *Public Health Reports, 100,* 131-146.

Larsson, K., & Ahlenius, S. (1999). Brain and sexual behavior. In J. G. McGinty (Ed.), Advancing from the ventral striatum to the extended amygdala: Implications for neuropsychiatry and drug abuse. *Annals of the New York Academy of Sciences, 877,* 292-308.

Larsson, L., Grimby, G., & Karlsson, J. (1979). Muscle strength and speed of movement in relation to age and muscle morphology. *Journal of Applied Physiology, 46(3)*, 451-456.

Lauterbur, P.C. (1973). Image formation by induced local interaction: Examples employing magnetic resonance. *Nature, 242*, 190-191.

Lawrence, R.H., & Jette, A.M. (1996). Disentangling the disablement process. *Journal of Gerontology: Social Sciences, 51B(4)*, S173-S182.

Lawton, M.P., & Nahemow, L. (1973). Ecology and the aging process. *Psychology of adult development and aging.* Washington, D.C.: American Psychological Association.

Leenders, K.L., Perani, D., Lammertsma, A.A., Heather, J.D., Buckingham, P., Healy, M.J.R., et al. (1990). Cerebral blood flow, blood volume and oxygen utilization. Normal values and effect of age. *Brain, 113*, 27-47.

Leger, L., & Thivierge, M. (1988). Heart rate monitors: Validity, stability, and functionality. *Physician & Sportsmedicine, 16*, 143-151

Lett, B.T., Grant, V.L., Koh, M.T., & Flynn, G. (2002). Prior experience with wheel running produces cross-tolerance to the rewarding effect of morphine. *Pharmacology, Biochemistry, & Behavior, 72 (1-2)*, 101-105.

Lewin, G.R., & Bard, Y.A. (1996). Physiology of the neurotrophins. *Annual Reviews in Neuroscience, 19*, 289-317.

Li, S.-C., & Lindenberger, U. (1999). Cross-level unification: A computational exploration of the link between deterioration of neurotransmitter systems and dedifferentiation of cognitive abilities in old age. In L.-G. Nillson and H.J. Markowitsch (Eds.), *Cognitive Neuroscience of Memory* (pp. 103-146). Seattle, WA: Hogrefe & Huber.

Liemohn, W.P. (1975). Strength and aging: An exploratory study. *Journal of Aging & Human Development, 6(4)*, 347-357.

Lifson, N., Gordon, G.B., Visscher, M.B., & Nier, A.O. (1949). The fate of utilized molecular oxygen and the source of heavy oxygen of respired carbon dioxide, studied with the aid of heavy oxygen. *Journal of Biological Chemistry, 180*, 803-811.

Lifson, N., Little, W.S., Levitt, D.G., & Henderson, R.M. (1975). $D_2{}^{18}O$ method for CO_2 output in small animals and economic feasibility in man. *Journal of Applied Physiology, 39*, 657-663.

Lifson, N., & McClintock, R. (1966). Theory of use of the turnover rates of body water for measuring energy and material balance. *Journal of Theoretical Biology, 12*, 46-74.

Lim, B.V., Jang, M.H., Shin, M.C., Kim, H.B., Kim, Y.J., Kim, Y.P., Chung, J.H., Kim, H., Shin, M.S., Kim, S.S., Kim, E.H., & Kim, C.J. (2001). Caffeine inhibits exercise-induced increase in tryptophan hydroxylase expression in dorsal and median raphe of Sprague-Dawley rats. *Neuroscience Letters, 308*, 25-28.

Liste, I., Guerra, M.J., Caruncho, H.J., & LabandeiraGarcia, J.L. (1997). Treadmill running induces striatal Fos expression via NMDA glutamate and dopamine receptors. *Experimental Brain Research, 115*, 458-468.

References

Lou, H.C., Edvinsson, L., & MacKenzie, E.T. (1987). The concept of coupling blood flow to brain function: Revision required? *Annals of Neurology, 22*, 289-297.

Louie, K., & Wilson, M.A. (2001). Temporally structured replay of awake hippocampal ensemble activity during rapid eye movement sleep. *Neuron, 29(1)*, 145-156.

Lowenthal, M.F., & Berkman, P.L. (1967). *Aging and mental disorder in San Francisco: A social psychiatric study.* San Francisco: Jossey-Bass.

Luskin, F.M., Newell, K.A., Griffith, M., Holmes, M., & Telles, S. (2000). A review of mind/body therapies in the treatment of musculoskeletal disorders with implications for the elderly. *Alternative Therapies in Health & Medicine, 6(2)*, 46-62.

Ma, Y.L., Wand, H.L., Wu, H.C., Wei, C.L., & Lee, E.H. (1998). Brain-derived neurotrophic factor antisense oligonucleotide impairs memory retention and inhibits long-term potentiation in rats. *Neuroscience, 82*, 957-967.

MacRae, P.G., Spirduso, W.W., Martin, T.P., Walters, T.J., Farrar, R.P., & Wilcox, R.E. (1987). Endurance training effects on striatal D2 dopamine receptor binding and striatal dopamine metabolites in presenescent older rats. *Psychopharmacology, 92*, 236-240.

Madden, D.J., Blumenthal, J.A., Allen, P.A., & Emery, C.F. (1989). Improving aerobic capacity in healthy older adults does not necessarily lead to improved cognitive performance. *Psychology & Aging, 4*, 307-320.

Madden, D.J., Turkington, T.G., Coleman, R.E., Provenzle, J.M., DeGrado, T.R., & Hoffman, J.M. (1996). Adult age differences in regional cerebral blood flow during visual word identification: Evidence from $H_2^{15}O$ PET. *NeuroImage, 3*, 127-142.

Madden, D.J., Turkington, T.G., Provenzale, J.M., Hawk, T.C., Hoffman, J.M., & Coleman, R.E. (1997). Selective and divided attention: Age-related changes in regional cerebral blood flow measured by H^{2-15O} PET. *Human Brain Mapping, 7*, 1115-1135.

Mahurin, R.K., DeBettignies, B.H., & Pirozzolo, F.J. (1991). Structured assessment of independent living skills: Preliminary report of a performance measure of functional abilities in dementia. *Journal of Gerontology: Psychological Sciences, 46(2)*, P58-P66.

Mamounas, L.A., Altar, C.A., Blue, M.E., Kaplan, D.R., Tessarollo, L., & Lyons, W.E. (2000). BDNF promotes the regenerative sprouting, but not survival, of injured serotonergic axons in the adult rat brain. *Journal of Neuroscience, 20*, 771-782

Manchanda, S.C., Narang, R., Reddy, K.S., Sachdeva, U., Prabhakaran, D., Dharmanand, S., Rajani, M., & Bijlani, R. (2000). Retardation of coronary atherosclerosis with yoga lifestyle intervention. *Journal of the Association of Physicians of India, 48(7)*, 687-94.

Mann, J. (1983). In S.T. McCarthy (Ed.), *Peripheral vascular disease in the elderly* (pp. 20-27). Edinburgh: Churchill Livingstone.

Manning, C.A., Parsons, M.W., & Gold, P.E. (1992). Anterograde and retrograde enhancement of 24-h memory by glucose in elderly humans. *Behavioral & Neural Biology, 58*, 125-130.

Manning, C.A., Stone, W.S., Korol, D.L., & Gold, P.E. (1998). Glucose enhancement of 24-h memory retrieval in healthy elderly humans. *Behavioural Brain Research, 93,* 71-76.

Manohcha, R., Marks, G.B., Kenchington, P., Peters, D., & Salome, C.M. (2002). Sahaja yoga in the management of moderate to severe asthma: A randomized controlled trial. *Thorax, 57(2),* 110-115.

Manson, J.E., Nathan, D.M., Sroleswski, A.S., Stampfer, M.J., Willett, W.C., & Hennekens, C.H. (1992). A prospective study of exercise and incidence of diabetes in U.S. male physicians. *Journal of the American Medical Association, 268,* 63-67.

Maquet, P. (2000). Functional neuroimaging of normal human sleep by positron emission tomography. *Journal of Sleep Research, 9(3),* 207-231.

Maquet, P., Laureys, S., Peigneux, P., Fuchs, S., Petiau, C., Phillips, C., Aerts, J., Del Fiore, G., Degueldre, C., Meulemans, T., Luxen, A., Franck, G., Van Der Linden, M., Smith, C., & Cleeremans, A. (2000). Experience-dependent changes in cerebral activation during human REM sleep. *Nature Neuroscience, 3(8),* 831-836.

Marchal, G.K., Rioux, P., Petit-Taboué, M.-C., Sette, G., Travére, J.-M., Le Poec, C., et al. (1992). Regional cerebral oxygen consumption, blood flow, and blood volume in healthy human aging. *Archives of Neurology, 49,* 1013-1020.

Marti, B., Pekkanen, J., Nissinen, A., Ketola, A., Kivela, S.L., Punsar, S., & Karvonen, M.J. (1989). Association of physical activity with coronary risk factors and physical ability: Twenty-year follow-up of a cohort of Finnish men. *Age & Ageing, 18,* 103-109.

Martin, A.J., Friston, K.J., Colebatch, J.G., & Frackowiak, R.S. (1991). Decreases in regional cerebral blood flow with normal aging. *Journal of Cerebral Blood Flow & Metabolism, 11,* 684-689.

Martin, W., Kohrt, W., Malley, M., Korte, K., & Stolz, S. (1990). Exercise training enhances leg vasodilatory capacity of 65-yr-old men and women. *Journal of Applied Physiology, 69,* 1804-1809.

Martinsen, E.W., & Morgan, W.P. (1997). Antidepressant effects of physical activity. In W.P. Morgan (Ed.), *Physical activity and mental health* (pp. 93-106). Washington, DC: Taylor & Francis.

Mather, A.S., Rodriguez, C., Guthrie, M.F., McHarg, A.M., Reid, I.C., & McMurdo, M.E. (2002). Effects of exercise on depressive symptoms in older adults with poorly responsive depressive disorder: Randomised controlled trial. *British Journal of Psychiatry, 180,* 411-415.

Mathes, W.F., & Kanarek, R.B. (2001). Wheel running attenuates the antinociceptive properties of morphine and its metabolite, morphine-6-glucuronide, in rats. *Physiology & Behavior, 74,* 245-251.

Mayr, U., Spieler, D.H., Kliegl, R. (Eds.). (2001). *Ageing and executive control.* Hove, East Sussex, England: Psychology Press, p. 303.

Mazzeo, R.S., Cavanagh, P., Evans, W.J., Fiatarone, M., Hagberg, J., McAuley, E., & Startzell, J. (1998). Exercise and physical activity for older adults: Position stand of the American College of Sports Medicine. *Medicine & Science in Sports & Exercise, 30(6),* 992-1008.

Mazziotta, J.C. (1989). Huntington's disease: Studies with structural imaging techniques and positron emission tomography. *Seminars in Neurology, 9,* 360-369.

Mazziotta, J.C., Frackowiak, R.S.J., & Phelps, M.E. (1992). The use of positron emission tomography in the clinical assessment of dementia. *Seminars in Nuclear Medicine, 22,* 233-246.

Mazziotta, J.C., Phelps, M.E., Pahl, J.J., Huang, S.C., Baxter, L.R., Riege, W.H., Hoffman, J.M., Kuhl, D.E., Lanto, A.B., Wapenski, J.A., et al. (1987). Reduced cerebral glucose metabolism in asymptomatic subjects at risk for Huntington's disease. *New England Journal of Medicine, 316,* 357-362.

Mazziotta, J.C., Phelps, M.E., Plummer, D. & Kuhl, D.E. (1981). Quantitation in positron emission tomography. Physical-anatomical effects. *Journal of Computer Assisted Tomography, 5,* 734-743.

Mazziotta, J., Toga, A., Evans, A., Fox, P., Lancaster, J., Zilles, K., et al. (2001). A probabilistic atlas and reference system for the human brain: International Consortium for Brain Mapping (ICBM). *Philosophical Transactions of the Royal Society of London Series B – Biological Sciences, 356,* 1293-1322.

Mazziotta, J.C., Toga, A.W., & Frackowiak, R.S.J. (Eds.) (2000). *Brain mapping: The disorders.* San Diego, CA: Academic Press.

McAllister, A.K., Katz, L.C., & Lo, D.C. (1999). Neurotrophins and synaptic plasticity. *Annual Reviews in Neuroscience, 22,* 295-318.

McArdle, W.D., Katch, F.L., & Katch, V.L. (1996). *Exercise physiology: Energy, nutrition, and human performance* (4th ed.). Baltimore: Williams & Wilkins.

McAulay, V., Deary, I.J., Ferguson, S.C., & Frier, B.M. (2001). Acute hypoglycemia in humans causes attentional dysfunction while nonverbal intelligence is preserved. *Diabetes Care, 10,* 1745-1750.

McAuley, E., & Rudolph, D. (1995). Physical activity, aging, and psychological well-being. *Journal of Aging & Physical Activity, 3(1),* 67-98.

McCloskey, D.P., Adamo, D.S., & Anderson, B.J. (2001). Exercise increases metabolic capacity in the motor cortex and striatum, but not in the hippocampus. *Brain Research, 891,* 168-175.

McCully, K., & Hamaoka, T. (2000). Near-infrared spectroscopy: What can it tell us about oxygen saturation in skeletal muscle? *Exercise Science Sport Reviews, 28,* 123-127.

McDowd, J.M., & Birren, J.E. (1990). Aging and attentional processes. In J.E. Birren & K.W. Schaie (Eds.), *Handbook of the psychology of aging* (pp. 222-230). New York: Academic Press.

McDowd, J.M., & Craik, F.I.M. (1988). Effects of aging and task difficulty on divided attention performance. *Journal of Experimental Psychology: Human Perception & Performance, 14,* 267-280.

McDowd, J.M., & Filion, D.L. (1992). Aging, selective attention, and inhibitory processes: A psychophysiological approach. *Psychology & Aging, 7,* 65-71.

References

McDowd, J.M., & Oseas-Kreger, D.M. (1991). Aging, inhibitory processes, and negative priming. *Journal of Gerontology: Psychological Sciences, 46*, P340-345.

McFarland, R.A. (1963). Experimental evidence of the relationship between aging and oxygen want: In search of a theory of aging. *Ergonomics, 6*, 339-366.

McFarland, R.A. (1968). The sensory and perceptual processes in aging. In K.W. Schaie (Ed.), *Theory and methods of research on aging* (pp. 9-52). Morgantown, WV: West Virginia University Press.

McGeer, P.L., Eccles, J.C., & McGeer, E.G. (1978). *Molecular neurobiology of the mammalian brain.* New York: Plenum Press.

McMorris, T., & Graydon, J. (2000). The effect of incremental exercise on cognitive performance. *International Journal of Sport Psychology, 31*, 66-81.

McNeil, J.K., LeBlanc, E.M., & Joyner, M. (1991). The effect of exercise on depressive symptoms in the moderately depressed elderly. *Psychology & Aging, 6(3)*, 487-488.

McPherson, B.D. (1990). *Aging as a social process.* Toronto: Butterworths.

McPherson, B.D. (1994). Sociocultural perspectives on aging and physical activity. *Journal of Aging & Physical Activity, 2,4*, 329-353.

Meeusen, R., Piacentini, M.F., Van Den Eynde, S., Magnus, L., & De Meirleir, K. (2001). Exercise performance is not influenced by a 5-HT reuptake inhibitor. *International Journal of Sports Medicine, 22*, 329-336.

Meeusen, R., Smolders, I., Saare, S., DeMeirleir, K., Keizer, H., Serneels, M., Ebinger, G., & Michotte Y. (1997). Endurance training effects on neurotransmitter release in rat striatum: An in vivo microdialysis study. *Acta Physiologica Scandinavica, 159*, 335-341.

Mega, M.S., Thompson, P.M., Toga, A.W., & Cummings, J.L. (2000). Brain mapping in dementia. In Mazziotta, J.C., Toga, A.W., & Frackowiak, R.S.J. (Eds.), *Brain mapping: The disorders* (pp. 217-239). San Diego: Academic Press.

Mehangoul-Schipper, D., Colier, W., & Jansen, R. (2001). Reproducibility of orthostatic changes in cerebral oxygenation in healthy subjects 70 years or older. *Clinical Physiology, 21*, 77-84.

Mehangoul-Schipper, J., Vloet, L., Colier, W., Hoefnagels, W., & Jansen, R. (2000). Cerebral oxgyenation declines in healthy elderly subjects in response to assuming the upright position. *Stroke, 31*, 1615-1620.

Melanson, E.L., Jr., & Freedson, P.S. (1995). Validity of the Computer Science and Applications, Inc. (CSA) activity monitor. *Medicine & Science in Sports & Exercise, 27*, 934-940.

Meltzer, C.C., Cantwell, M.N., Greer, P.J., Ben-Eliezer, D., Smith, G., Frank, G., et al. (2000). Does cerebral blood flow decline in healthy aging? A PET study with partial-volume correction. *Journal of Nuclear Medicine, 41*, 1842-1848.

Messier, C., Durkin, T., Mrabet, O., & Destrade, C. (1990). Memory-improving action of glucose: Indirect evidence for a facilitation of hippocampal acetylcholine synthesis. *Behavioural Brain Research, 39*, 135-143.

Meyer, J.S., Obara, K., & Muramatsu, K. (1993). Diaschisis. *Neurology Research, 15*, 362-366.

References

Meyer, J.S., Terayama, Y., & Takashima, S. (1993). Cerebral circulation in the elderly. *Cerebrovascular & Brain Metabolism Reviews, 5*, 122-146.

Meyer, J.S., Welch, K.M.A., Titus, J.L., Suzuki, M., Kim, H.S., Perez, F.I., et al. (Eds.). (1976). *Neurotransmitter failure in cerebral infarction and dementia*. New York: Raven Press.

Miller, A.K.H., Alston, R.L., & Corsellis, J.A.N. (1980). Variation with age in the volumes of grey and white matter in the cerebral hemispheres of man— Measurements with an image analyzer. *Neuropathology and Applied Neurobiology, 6*, 119-132.

Miller, L.S., Bedwell, J.S., Allison, J., & Strauss, G. (2002). A robust, qualitatively similar but quantitatively different BOLD response in healthy older versus younger adults on a retinal photic-stimulation task [Abstract]. *Biological Psychiatry, 51*, 196S.

Miller, S., Bedwell, J., Yanasak, N., Allison, J. (2003). Age effects on the Stroop Color-Word task as measured by the fMRI BOLD response [Abstract]. *Journal of the International Neuropsychological Society, 9*, 137.

Miszko, T.A., Cress, M.E., Slade, J.M., Covey, C.J., Agrawal, S.K., & Doerr, C.E. (2003). Effect of strength and power training on physical function in community-dwelling older adults. *Journal of Gerontology: Medical Science, 58(2)*, M171-175.

Mitchell, D.G., & Cohen, M. (2004). *MRI Principles* (2nd ed.). New York: W. B. Saunders, Elsevier.

Mitrushina, M., & Satz, P. (1991). Analysis of longitudinal covariance structures in assessment of stability of cognitive functions in elderly. *Brain Dysfunction, 4*, 163-173.

Mobily, K.E., Rubenstein, L.M., Lemke, J.H., O'Hara, M.W., & Wallace, R.B. (1996). Walking and depression in a cohort of older adults: The Iowa 65+ rural health study. *Journal of Aging & Physical Activity, 4(2)*, 119-135.

Moldofsky, H., Lue, F., & Smythe, H. (1983). Alpha EEG sleep and morning symptoms in rheumatic arthritis. *Journal of Rheumatology, 10*, 373-379.

Mondadori, C., & Petschke, F. (1987). Do piracetam-like compounds act centrally via peripheral mechanisms? *Brain Research, 435*, 310-314.

Montoye, H.J. (1975). *Physical activity and health: An epidemiologic study of an entire community*. Englewood Cliffs, NJ: Prentice Hall.

Montoye, H.J., Kemper, H.C.G., Saris, W.H.M., & Washburn, R.A. (1996). *Measuring physical activity and energy expenditure*. Champaign, IL: Human Kinetics.

Montoye, H.J., Servais, S.B., & Webster, J.G. (1986). Estimation of energy expenditure from a force platform and an accelerometer. In J. Watkins, T. Reilly, & L. Burwitz (Eds.), *Sport science* (pp. 375-380). London: E. & F.N. Spoon.

Montoye, H.J., & Taylor, H.L. (1984). Measurement of physical activity in population studies: A Review. *Human Biology, 56*, 195-216.

Moraska, A., & Fleshner, M. (2001). Voluntary physical activity prevents stress-induced behavioral depression and anti-KLH antibody suppression. *American*

Journal of Physiology—Regulatory Interactive and Comparative Physiology, 281(2), R484-R489.

Morey, M.C., Schenkman, M., Studenski, S.A., Chandler, J.M., Crowley, G.M., Sullivan, R.J., Pieper, C.F., Doyle, M.E., Higginbotham, M.B., Horner, R.D., MacAller, H., Puglisi, C. M., Morris, K.G., & Weinberger, M. (1999). Spinal flexibility plus aerobic versus aerobic only training: Effects of a randomized clinical trial on function in at risk older adults. *Journal of Gerontology: Medical Sciences, 54A(7),* M335-M342.

Morgan, W.P. (1997). *Physical activity and mental health.* Washington, DC: Taylor & Francis.

Moss, M.C., & Scholey, A.B. (1996). Oxygen administration enhances memory formation in healthy young adults. *Psychopharmacology, 124,* 255-260.

Moss, M.C., Scholey, A.B., & Wesnes, K. (1998). Oxygen administration selectively enhances cognitive performance in healthy young adults: A placebo-controlled double-blind crossover study. *Psychopharmacology, 138,* 27-33.

Moul, J.L., Goldman, B., & Warren, B. (1995). Physical activity and cognitive performance in the older population. *Journal of Aging & Physical Activity, 3,* 135-145.

Mufson, E.J., Kroin, J.S., Sendera, T.J., & Sobreviela, T. (1999). Distribution and retrograde transport of trophic factors in the central nervous system: Functional implications for the treatment of neurodegenerative diseases. *Progress in Neurobiology, 57,* 451-484.

Müller-Gärtner, H.W., Links, J.M., Prince, J.L., Bryan, R.N., McVeigh, E., Leal, J.P., Davatzikos, C., & Frost, J.J. (1992). Measurement of radiotracer concentration in brain gray matter using positron emission tomography: MRI-based correction for partial volume effects. *Journal of Cerebral Blood Flow & Metabolism, 12,* 571-583.

Myers, J.K., Weissman, M.M., Tischler, G.L., Holzer, C.E. 3rd, Leaf, P.J., Orvaschel, H., Anthony, J.C., & Boyd, J.H. (1984). Six-month prevalence of psychiatric disorders in three communities 1980 to 1982. *Archives of General Psychiatry, 41(10),* 959-967.

Myerson, J., Hale, S., Wagstaff, D., Poon, L.W., & Smith, G.A. (1990). The information-loss model: A mathematical theory of age-related cognitive slowing. *Psychological Review, 97(4),* 475-487.

Nagai, Y., Kemper, M., Earley, C., & Metter, E. (1998). Blood flow velocities and their relationships in carotid and middle cerebral arteries. *Ultrasound in Medicine & Biology, 24,* 1131-1136.

Nagi, S.Z. (1976). An epidemiology of disability among adults in the United States. *Milbank Memorial Fund Quarterly, 54,* 439-467.

Nagi, S.Z. (1991). Disability concepts revisited: Implications for prevention. In A.M. Pope & A.R. Tarlov (Eds.). *Disability in America: Toward a national agenda for prevention* (pp. 309-327). Washington, D.C.: National Academy Press.

Nakken, K. (1999). Physical exercise in outpatients with epilepsy. *Epilepsia, 40,* 643-651.

Nakken, K.O., Bjorholt, P.G., Johannessen, S.I., Loyning, T., & Lind, E. (1990). Effect of physical training on aerobic capacity, seizure occurrence, and serum level of antiepileptic drugs in adults with epilepsy. *Epilepsia, 31,* 88-94.

References

Naylor, E., Penev, P.D., Orbeta, L., Janssen, I., Ortiz, R., Colecchia, E.F., Keng, M., Finkel, S., & Zee, P.C. (2000). Daily social and physical activity increases slow-wave sleep and daytime neuropsychological performance in the elderly. *Sleep, 23(1),* 87-95.

Nebes, R.D., & Madden, D.J. (1988). Different patterns of cognitive slowing produced by Alzheimer's disease and normal aging. *Psychology & Aging, 3,* 102-104.

Neeper, S.A., Gomez-Pinilla, F., Choi, J., & Cotman, C. (1995). Exercise and brain neurotrophins. *Nature, 373,* 109.

Neeper, S.A., Gomez-Pinilla, F., Choi, J., & Cotman, C.W. (1996). Physical activity increases mRNA for brain-derived neurotrophic factor and nerve growth factor in rat brain. *Brain Research, 726,* 49-56.

Niedermeyer, E. (Ed.). (1987). *EEG and old age.* Baltimore: Urban & Schwarzenberg.

Nielsen, H.B., Boesen, M., & Secher, N.H. (2001). Near-infrared spectroscopy determined brain and muscle oxygenation during exercise with normal and resistive breathing. *Acta Physiologica Scandanavica, 171,* 63-70.

Nielsen, H.B., Boushel, R., Madsen, P., & Secher, N.H. (1999). Cerebral desaturation during exercise reversed by O_2 supplementation. *American Journal of Physiology, 277,* H1045-H1052.

Nieman, D.C., Henson, D.A., Gusewitch, G., Warren, B.J., Dotson, R.C., Butterworth, D.E., & Nehlsen-Cannarella, S.L. (1993). Physical activity and immune function in elderly women. *Medicine & Science in Sports & Exercise, 25,* 823-831.

Nikiforova, A.S., Patchev, V.K., & Nikolov, N.D. (1989). Long-term locomotion regimens affect EEG paroxysmal activity, behaviour and sex hormone secretion in female rats. *Acta Physiologica et Pharmacologica Bulgarica, 15,* 31-37.

Nikiforova, A.S., Patchev, V.K., Nikolov, N.D., & Cheresharov, L. (1988). Spontaneous EEG paroxysmal activity and behavior in female rats subjected to running exercise or to physiological restriction of the locomotion. *Activitas Nervosa Superior (Praha), 30,* 233-234.

Nitzke, R.W. (1971). *The life of Wilhelm Conrad Roentgen, discoverer of the X-ray.* Tucson, AZ: University of Arizona Press.

North, T.C., McCullagh, P., & Tran, Z.V. (1990). Effect of exercise on depression. *Exercise & Sport Sciences Reviews, 18,* 379-416.

Obrig, H., Hirth, C., Junge-Hulsing, J.G., Doge, C., Wolf, T., Dirnagl, U., & Villringer, A. (1996). Cerebral oxygenation changes in response to motor stimulation. *Journal of Applied Physiology, 81,* 1174-1183.

Obrig, H., & Villringer, A. (1997). Near-infrared spectroscopy in functional activation studies: Can NIRS demonstrate cortical activation? In A. Villringer, & U. Dirnagl (Eds.), *Optical imaging of brain function and metabolism* (pp. 113-127). New York: Plenum Press.

O'Connor, P.J. (1997). Overtraining and staleness. In W.P. Morgan (Ed.), *Physical activity and mental health* (pp. 145-159). Washington, DC: Taylor & Francis.

References

O'Connor, P.J., Aenchbacher, L.E., & Dishman, R.K. (1995). Physical Activity and depression in the elderly. *Journal of Aging & Physical Activity, 1(1)*, 34-58.

Ogawa, S., Lee, T.M., Nayak, A.S., & Glynn, P. (1990). Oxygenation-sensitive contrast in magnetic-resonance image of rodent brain at high magnetic fields. *Magnetic Resonance Medicine, 14*, 68-78.

Ogawa, S., Menon, R.S., Tank, D.W., Kim, S.G., Merkle, H., Ellermann, J.M., et al., (1993). Functional brain mapping by blood oxygenation level-dependent contrast magnetic-resonance imaging: A comparison of signal characteristics with a biophysical model. *Biophysics Journal, 64*, 803-812.

O'Grady, M., & Wolf, S.L. (2002). A critical review of tai chi chuan. In S. Wainapel and A. Fast (Eds.), *Alternative medicine in rehabilitation*. New York: Demos Press.

Oliff, H.S., Berchtold, N.C., Isackson, P., & Cotman, C.W. (1998). Exercise-induced regulation of brain-derived neurotrophic factor (BDNF) transcripts in the rat hippocampus. *Molecular Brain Research, 61*, 147-153.

Olive, J., DeVan, A., & McCully, K. (2002). The effects of aging and activity on muscle blood flow. *Dynamic Med, 1*, 2.

Olsen, H., & Lanne, T. (1998). Reduced venous compliance in lower limbs of aging humans and its importance for capacitance function. *American Journal of Physiology: Heart Circulation, 44*, H878-H886.

O'Neal, H.A., Van Hoomissen, J.D., Holmes, P.V., & Dishman, R.K. (2001). Prepro-galanin messenger RNA levels are increased in rat locus coeruleus after treadmill exercise training. *Neuroscience Letters, 299(1-2)*, 69-72

Ostir, G.V., Markides, K.S., Black, S.A., & Goodwin, J.S. (1998). Lower-body functioning as a predictor of subsequent disability among older Mexican Americans. *Journal of Gerontology: Medical Sciences, 53A(6)*, M491-M495.

Ouellet, D., & Moffett, H. (2002). Locomotor deficits before and two months after knee arthroplasty. *Arthritis & Rheumatism, 47(5)*, 484-493.

Overall, J.E., & Gorham, D.R. (1972). Organicity versus old age in objective and projective test performance. *Journal of Consulting Clinical Psychology, 39*, 98-105.

Owler, B., & Pickard, J. (2001). Normal pressure hydrocephalus and cerebral blood flow: A review. *Acta Neurologica Scandinavica, 104*, 325-342.

Paffenbarger, R.S. Jr., Blair, S.N., Lee, I.M., & Hyde, R.T. (1993). Measurement of physical activity to assess health effects in free-living populations. *Medicine & Science in Sports & Exercise, 25*, 60-70.

Pantano, P. Baron, J.C., Lebrun-Grandie, P., Duquesnoy, N., Bousser, M.G., & Comar, D. (1984). Regional cerebral blood flow and oxygen consumption in human aging. *Stroke, 15*, 635-641.

Panton, L.B., Graves, J.E., Pollock, M.L., Hagberg, J.M., & Chen, W. (1990). Effect of aerobic and resistance training on fractionated reaction time and speed of movement. *Journal of Gerontology, 45*, M26-31.

Papadakis, M.A., Grady, D., Black, D., Tierney, M.J., Gooding, G.A.W., Schambelan, M., & Grunfeld, C. (1996). Growth hormone replacement in healthy older men improves body composition but not functional ability. *Annals of Internal Medicine, 124*, 708-716.

Park, R.J. (1992). Human energy expenditure from Australopithecus afarensis to the 4-minute mile: Exemplars and case studies. *Exercise & Sport Sciences Reviews, 20*, 185-220.

Patrick, G.T., & Gilbert, J.A. (1896). On the effects of loss of sleep. *Psychological Review, 3*, 469-483.

Paus, T. (2001). Primate anterior cingulate cortex: Where motor control, drive and cognition interface. *Nature Reviews Neuroscience, 2(6)*, 417-424.

Pereira, M.A., Fitzgerald, S.J., Gregg, E.W., Joswiak, M.L., Ryan, W.J., Suminski, R.R., Utter, A.C., & Zmuda, J.M. (1997). A collection of physical questionnaires for health-related research. *Medicine & Science in Sports & Exercise, 29(6)*, S03-S205.

Perret, R.S., & Sloop, G.D. (2000). Increased peak blood velocity in association with elevated blood pressure. *Ultrasound in Medicine & Biology, 26(9)*, 1387-1391.

Perusse, L., Tremblay, A., LeBlanc, C., & Bouchard, C. (1989). Genetic and familial environmental influences on level of habitual physical activity. *American Journal of Epidemiology, 129*, 1012-1022.

Petrella, J.K., Miller, L.S., & Cress, M.E. (2004). Leg extensor power, cognition, and functional performance in independent and marginally dependent older adults. *Age & Ageing, 33*, 1-7.

Petruzzello, S.J., Landers, D.M., Hatfield, B.D., Kubitz, K.A., & Salazar, W. (1991). A meta-analysis on the anxiety reducing effects of acute and chronic exercise, *Sports Medicine, 11*, 143-182.

Pfefferbaum, A., Mathalon, D.H., Sullivan, E.V., Rawles, J.M., Zipursky, R.B., & Lim, K.O. (1994). A quantitative magnetic resonance imaging study of changes in brain morphology from infancy to late adulthood. *Archives of neurology, 51(9)*, 874-887.

Plante, T.G., & Rodin, J. (1990). Physical fitness and enhanced psychological health. *Current Psychology: Research & Reviews, 9*, 3-24.

Plude, D.J., & Hoyer, W.J. (1985). Attention and performance: Identifying and localizing age deficits. In N. Charness (Ed.), *Aging and performance* (pp. 47-99). New York: Wiley.

Podsiadlo, D., & Richardson, S. (1991). The timed 'up & go': A test of basic functional mobility for frail elderly persons. *Journal of the American Geriatrics Society, 39*, 142-148.

Poehlman, E., Gardner, A., Goran, M., Arciero, P., Toth, M., Ades, P., & Calles-Escandon, J. (1995). Sympathetic nervous system activity, body fatness, and body fat distribution in younger and older males. *Journal of Applied Physiology, 78*, 802-806.

Pollard, V., Prough, D.S., DeMelo, A.E., Deyo, D.J., Uchida, T., & Stoddart, H.F. (1996). Validation in volunteers of a near infrared spectroscope for monitoring brain oxygenation in vivo. *Anesthesia & Analgesia, 82*, 269-277.

Pollock, M.L., Gaesser, G.A., Butcher, J.D., Despres, J.P., Dishman, R.K., Franklin, B.A., & Garber, C.E. (1998). Recommended quantity and quality of exercise for developing and maintaining cardiorespiratory and muscular fitness, and flexibility in healthy adults. *Medicine & Science in Sports & Exercise, 30,* 975-991.

Poon, L.W. (Ed.). (1980). *Aging in the 1980s; Psychological issues.* Washington, DC: American Psychological Assoc.

Poon, L.W. (1985). Differences in human memory with aging: Nature, causes, and clinical implications. In J.E. Birren & K.W. Shaie (Eds.), *Handbook of the psychology of aging,* 2nd ed. (xvii, pp. 427-462). New York: Van Nostrand Reinhold.

Poon, L.W. (1993). Assessing neuropsychological changes in pharmacological trials. *Clinical Neuropharmacology, 16,* S31-S38.

Poon, L.W., Rubin, D.C., & Wilson, B.A. (Eds.). (1989). *Everyday cognition in adulthood and late life.* New York: Cambridge University Press.

Prentice, A.M. (Ed.). (1990). *The doubly-labeled water method for measuring energy expenditure: A consensus report by the IDECG working group technical recommendations for use in humans.* Vienna, Austria: International Dietary Energy Consultancy Group, International Atomic Energy Agency, Section of Nutritional and Health-Related Environmental Studies.

Prinz, P.N., Dustman, R.E., & Emmerson, R.Y. (1990). Electrophysiology and aging. In J.E. Birren, & K.W. Schaie (Eds.), *Handbook of the psychology of aging* (3rd ed., pp. 135-149). San Diego: Academic Press.

Proctor, D., Shen, P., Dietz, N., Eickhoff, T., Lawler, L., Ebersold, E., Loeffler, D., & Joyner, M. (1998). Reduced leg blood flow during dynamic exercise in older endurance-trained men. *Journal of Applied Physiology, 85(1),* 68-75.

Province, M.A., Hadley, E.C., Hornbrook, M.C., Lipsitz, L.A., Miller, J.P., Mulrow, C.D., Ory, M.G., Sattin, R.W., Tinetti, M.E., & Wolf, S.L. (1995). The effects of exercise on falls in elderly patients: A preplanned meta-analysis of the FICSIT trials. *Journal of the American Medical Association, 273,* 1341-1347.

Quaresima, V., Colier, W., Sluijs, M., & Ferrari, M. (2001). Nonuniform quadriceps O_2 consumption revealed by near infrared multipoint measurements. *Biochemical & Biophysical Research Communications, 285,* 1034-1039.

Radak, Z., Kaneko, T., Tahara, S., Nakamoto, H., Pucsok, J., Sasvari, M., Nyakas, C., & Goto, S. (2001). Regular exercise improves cognitive function and decreases oxidative damage in rat brain. *Neurochemistry International, 38,* 17-23.

Raglin, J.S. (1997). Anxiolytic effects of physical activity. In W.P. Morgan (Ed.), *Physical activity and mental health* (pp. 107-127). Washington, DC: Taylor & Francis.

Rajala, U., Uusimaki, A., Keinanen-Kiukaanniemi, S., & Kivela, S.L. (1994). Prevalence of depression in a 55-year-old Finnish population. *Social Psychiatry & Psychiatric Epidemiology, 29(3),* 126-130.

Rajkowska, G. (2000). Postmortem studies in mood disorders indicate altered numbers of neurons and glial cells. *Biological Psychiatry, 48,* 766-777.

Rankin, J.K., Woollacot, M.H., Shumway-Cook, A., & Brown, L.A. (2000). Cognitive influence on postural stability: A neuromuscular analysis in young and older adults. *Journal of Gerontology: Medical Sciences, 55A(3),* M112-M119.

References

Raz, N., Gunning, F.M., Head, D., Dupuis, J.H., McQuain, J., Briggs, S.D., Loken, W.J., Thornton, A.E., & Acker, J.D. (1997). Selective aging of the human cerebral cortex observed in vivo: Differential vulnerability of the prefrontal gray matter. *Cerebral Cortex, 7(3)*, 268-282.

Regan, D. (1972). *Evoked potentials in psychology: Sensory physiology and clinical medicine*. London: Chapman & Hall.

Reiman, E.M., Caselli, R.J., Yn, L.S., Chen, K., Bandy, D., Minoshima, S., Thibodeau, S.N., & Osborne, D. (1996). Preclinical evidence of Alzheimer's disease in persons homozygous for the epsilon 4 allele for apolipoprotein. E. *New England Journal of Medicine, 334*, 752-758.

Reuben, D.B. (1991). *Geriatric syndromes* (2nd ed., pp. 117-231). New York: American Geriatrics Society.

Reuben, D.B., Frank, J.C., Hirsch, S.H., McGuigan, K.A., & Maly, R.C. (1999). A randomized clinical trial of outpatient comprehensive geriatric assessment coupled with an intervention to increase adherence to recommendations. *Journal of the American Geriatrics Society, 47*, 269-276.

Reuben, D.B., Siu, A.L., & Kimpau, S. (1992). The predictive validity of self-report and performance-based measures of function and health. *Journal of Gerontology: Medical Sciences, 47(4)*, M106-M110.

Reuter-Lorenz, P.A., Jonides, J., Smith, E.E., Harley, A., Miller, A. Marshuetz, C., & Koeppe, R. (2000). Age differences in the frontal lateralization of verbal and spatial working memory revealed by PET. *Journal of Cognitive Neuroscience, 12*, 174-187.

Richter, E.A., & Sutton, J.A. (1994). Hormonal adaptations to physical activity. In C. Bouchard, R.J. Shephard, & T. Stephens (Eds.), *Physical activity, fitness and health: International proceedings and consensus statement*. Champaign, IL: Human Kinetics, pp. 331-342.

Rikli, R., & Busch, S. (1986). Motor performance of women as a function of age and physical activity level. *Journal of Gerontology, 41 (5)*, 645-649.

Rikli, R.F., & Jones, C.J. (1999). Development and validation of a functional fitness test for community-residing older adults. *Journal of Aging & Physical Activity, 7*, 129-161.

Roberts, D., Bolinger, L., Detre, J., Insk, E., Bergey, P., & Leigh, J. (1993). Continuous inversion angiography. *Magnetic Resonance Medicine, 29*, 631-636.

Roberts, E. (1972). Coordination between excitation and inhibition: Development of the GABA system. In C.D. Clemente, D.P. Purpura, & F.E. Mayer (Eds.), *Sleep and the maturing nervous system* (pp. 79-97). New York: Academic Press.

Roberts, S.B., Dietz, W., Sharp, T., Dallal, G.E., & Hill, J. (1995). Multiple laboratory comparison of the doubly labeled water technique. *Obesity Research, 3(Suppl. 1)*, 3-13.

Rogers, R.L., Meyer, J.S., & Mortel, K.F. (1990). After reaching retirement age physical activity sustains cerebral perfusion and cognition. *Journal of the American Geriatrics Society, 38*, 123-128.

Rombouts, S.A., Barkhof, F., Witter, M.P., & Scheltens, P. (2000). Unbiased whole-brain analysis of gray matter loss in Alzheimer's disease. *Neuroscience Letters, 285*, 231-233.

References

Rosen, A.C., Prull, M.W., O'Hara, R., Race, E.A., Desmond, J.E., Glover, G.H., Yesavage, J.A., & Gabrieli, J.D. (2002). Variable effects of aging on frontal lobe contributions to memory. *Neuroreport, 13,* 2425-2428.

Rosenzweig, M.R., & Bennett, E.L. (1996). Psychobiology of plasticity: Effects of training and experience on brain and behavior. *Behavioural Brain Research, 78,* 57-65.

Rossitier-Fornoff, J.E., Wolf, S.L., Wolfson, L.I., & Buchner, D.M. (1995). A cross-sectional validation study of the FICSIT common database balance measures. Frailty and Injuries: Cooperative Studies of Intervention Techniques. *Journal Gerontology: Medical Sciences, 50(6),* M291-M297.

Roth, R.H., & Elsworth, J.D. (1995). Biochemical pharmacology of midbrain dopamine neurons. In F.E. Bloom & D.J. Kupfer (Eds.), *Psychopharmacology: The fourth generation of progress* (pp. 227-243). New York: Raven Press.

Rowe, J.W., & Kahn, R.L. (1987). Human aging: Usual and successful. *Science, 237,* 143-149.

Rowe, J.W., & Kahn, R.L. (1998). *Successful aging.* New York: Dell.

Roy, C.W., & Sherrington, C.S. (1890). On the regulation of the blood supply of the brain. *Journal of Physiology (London), 11,* 85-108.

Royall, D.R., Palmer, R., Chiodo, L.K., & Polk, M.J. (2004). Declining executive control in normal aging predicts change in functional status: The Freedom House Study. *Journal of the American Geriatrics Society, 54(3),* 346-352.

Russo-Neustadt, A., Beard, R.C., & Cotman, C.W. (1999). Exercise, anti-depressant medications and enhanced neurotrophic factor expression. *Neuropsychopharmacology, 21,* 679-682.

Russo-Neustadt, A., Ha, T., Ramirez, R., & Kesslak, J.P. (2001). Physical activity-antidepressant treatment combination: Impact on brain-derived neurotrophic factor and behavior in an animal model. *Behavioral Brain Research, 120,* 87-95.

Saito, S., Nishihara, F., Takazawa, T., Kanai, M., Aso, C., Shiga, T., & Shimada, H. (1999). Exercise-induced cerebral deoxygenation among untrained trekkers at moderate altitudes. *Archives of Environmental Health, 54,* 271-276.

Saitou, H., Yanagi, H., Hara, S., Tsuchiya, S., & Tomura, S. (2000). Cerebral blood volume and oxgyenation among poststroke hemiplegic patients: Effects of 13 rehabilitation tasks measured by near-infrared spectroscopy. *Archives of Physical Medicine Rehabilitation, 81,* 1348-1356.

Sallis, J.F., & Saelens, B.E. (2000). Assessment of physical activity by self-report: Status, limitations, and future directions. *Research Quarterly for Exercise & Sport, 71,* 1-14.

Salmon, E., & Franck, G. (1989). Positron emission tomographic study in Alzheimer's disease and Pick's disease. *Archives of Gerontology & Geriatrics, 1,* 241-247.

Salthouse, T.A. (1985). Speed of behavior and its implications for cognition. In J.E. Birren, & K.W. Schaie (Eds.), *Handbook of the psychology of aging* (2nd ed,). (pp. 400-426). New York: Van Nostrand Reinhold.

Salthouse, T.A. (1988). Resource-reduction interpretations of cognitive aging. *Developmental Review, 8,* 238-272.

References

Salthouse, T.A. (1992). *Mechanisms of age-cognition relations in adulthood.* Hillsdale, NH: Lawrence Erlbaum.

Salthouse, T.A. (1997). The processing speed theory of adult age differences in cognition. *Psychological Review, 103,* 403-429.

Salthouse, T.A. (1999). Cognitive and information-processing perspectives on aging. In I.H. Nordhus, G.R. VandenBos, S. Berg, & P. Gromholr (Eds.), *Clinical Geropsychology.* Washington, DC: American Psychological Assoc.

Salthouse, T.A., Rogan, J.D., & Prill, K. (1984). Division of attention: Age differences on a visually presented memory task. *Memory & Cognition, 12,* 613-620.

Samorajski, T., Rolsten, C., Przykorska, A., & Davis, C.M. (1987). Voluntary wheel running exercise and monoamine levels in brain, heart and adrenal glands of aging mice. *Experimental Gerontology, 22,* 421-431.

Sanders-Bush, E., & Canton, H. (1995). Serotonin receptors: Signal transduction pathways. In F.E. Bloom, & D.J. Kupfer (Eds.), *Psychopharmacology: The fourth generation of progress.* New York: Raven Press, pp. 431-441.

Sato, R., Bryan, R.N., & Fried, L.P. (1999). Neuroanatomic and functional correlates of depressed mood: The Cardiovascular Health Study. *American Journal of Epidemiology, 150(9),* 919-929.

Savin, E., Siegelova, J., Fisher, B., & Bonnin, P. (1997). Intra- and extracranial artery blood velocity during a sudden blood pressure decrease in humans. *European Journal of Applied Physiology, 76,* 289-293.

Schaie, K.W. (1989). The hazards of cognitive aging. *Gerontologist, 29,* 484-493.

Schechtman, K.B., Kutner, N.G., Wallace, R.B., Buchner, D.M., & Ory, M.G. (1997). Gender, self-reported depressive symptoms, and sleep disturbance among older community-dwelling persons. FICSIT group. Frailty and Injuries: Cooperative Studies of Intervention Techniques. *Journal of Psychosomatic Research, 43(5),* 513-527.

Scheel, P., Ruge, C., Petruch, U., & Schoning, M. (2000). Color duplex measurement of cerebral blood flow volume in healthy adults. *Stroke, 31,* 147-150.

Scheel, P., Ruge, C., & Schoning, M. (2000). Flow velocity and flow volume measurements in the extracranial carotid and vertebral arteries in healthy adults: Reference data and the effects of age. *Ultrasound in Medicine & Biology, 26,* 1261-1266.

Schenkenberg, T. (1970). Visual, auditory, and somatosensory, evoked responses of normal subjects from childhood to senescence. (Unpublished doctoral dissertation, University of Utah, 1970).

Schoeller, D.A. (1988). Measurement of energy expenditure in free-living humans using doubly labeled water. *Journal of Nutrition, 118,* 1278-1289.

Schoeller, D.A. (1999). Recent advances from application of doubly labeled water to measurement of human energy expenditure. *Journal of Nutrition, 129,* 1765-1768.

Schoeller, D.A., & van Santen, E. (1982). Measurement of energy expenditure in humans by doubly-labelled water method. *Journal of Applied Physiology, 53,* 955-959.

References

Scholey, A.B., Harper, S., & Kennedy, D.O. (2001). Cognitive demand and blood glucose. *Physiology & Behavior, 73,* 585-592.

Scholey, A.B., Moss, M.C., Neave, N., & Wesnes, K. (1999). Cognitive performance, hyperoxia, and heart rate following oxygen administration in healthy young adults. *Physiology & Behavior, 67,* 783-789.

Scholey, A.B., Moss, M.C., & Wesnes, K. (1998). Oxygen and cognitive performance: The temporal relationship between hyperoxia and enhanced memory. *Psychopharmacology, 140,* 123-126.

Scudds, R.J., & Ostbye, T. (2001). Pain and pain-related interference with function in older Canadians: The Canadian Study of Health and Aging. *Disability & Rehabilitation, 23(15),* 654-664.

Seal, L.J., Small, C.J., Kim, M.S., et al. (2000). Prolactin releasing peptide (PrRP) stimulates luteinizing hormone (LH) and follicle stimulating hormone (FSH) via a hypothalamic mechanism in male rats. *Endocrinology, 141,* 1909–1912.

Seeman, P. (1995). Dopamine receptors clinical correlates. In F.E. Bloom & D.J. Kupfer (Eds.), *Psychopharmacology: The fourth generation of progress* (pp. 295-302). New York: Raven Press.

Seidel, E., Eicke, B., Tettenborn, B., & Kurummenauer, F. (1999). Reference values for vertebral artery flow volume by duplex sonography in young and elderly adults. *Stroke, 30,* 2692-2696.

Shephard, R.J., & Leith, L.M. (1990). Physical activity and cognitive changes with aging. In M.L. Howe, M.J. Stones, & D.C.J. Brainer (Eds.), *Cognitive and behavioral performance factors in atypical aging* (pp. 154-180). New York: Springer.

Sherwood, D.E., & Selder, D.J. (1979). Cardiorespiratory health, reaction time and aging. *Medicine & Science in Sports & Exercise, 11,* 186-189.

Shirayama, Y., Chen, A.C.-H., Nakagawa, S., Russell, D.S., & Duman, R.S. (2002). Brain-derived neurotrophic factor produces antidepressant effects in behavioral models of depression. *Journal of Neuroscience, 22,* 3251-3261.

Siconolfi, S.F., Lasater, T.M., Snow, R.C.K., & Carleton, R.A. (1985). Self-reported physical activity compared with maximal oxygen uptake. *American Journal of Epidemiology, 122,* 101-105.

Silver, I.A. (1978). Cellular microenvironment in relation to local blood flow. In K. Elliot & M. O'Connor (Eds.), *Cerebral vascular smooth muscle and its control* (pp. 49-61). New York: Elsevier.

Simonson, S.G., & Piantidosi, C.A. (1996). Near-infrared spectroscopy: Clinical applications. *Critical Care Clinics, 12,* 1019-1029.

Singh, M.A.F. (2002). Exercise comes of age: Rationale and recommendations for a geriatric exercises prescription. *Journal of Gerontology: Medical Sciences, 57A(5),* M262-M282.

Singh, N.A., Clements, K.M., & Fiatarone, M.A. (1997). A randomized controlled trial of the effect of exercise on sleep. *Sleep, 20(2),* 95-101.

Singh, N.A., Clements, K.M., & Singh, M.A. (2001). The efficacy of exercise as a long-term antidepressant in elderly subjects: A randomized, controlled trial. *Journal of Gerontology: Biological Science & Medical Science, 56A(8),* M497-504.

Sisti, H.M., & Lewis, M.J. (2001). Naloxone suppression and morphine enhancement of voluntary wheel-running activity in rats. *Pharmacology, Biochemistry, & Behavior, 70*, 359-365.

Siuciak, J.A., Lewis, D.R., Wiegand, S.J., & Lindsay, R.M. (1997). Antidepressant-like effect of brain-derived neurotrophic factor (BDNF). *Pharmacology, Biochemistry, & Behavior, 56*, 131-137.

Skalicky, M., Bubna-Littitz, H., & Vidiik, A. (1996). Influence of physical exercise on aging rats: I. Life-long exercise preserves patterns of spontaneous activity. *Mechanisms of Ageing & Development, 87*, 127-139.

Slosman, D.O., Chicherio, C., Ludwig, C., Genton, L., de Ribaupierre, S., Hans, D., et al. (2001). ^{133}Xe SPECT cerebral blood flow study in a healthy population: Determination of T-scores. *Journal of Nuclear Medicine, 42*, 864-870.

Small, S.A., Nava, A.S., Perera, G.M., Delapaz, R., & Stern, Y. (2000). Evaluating the function of hippocampal subregions with high-resolution MRI in Alzheimer's disease and aging. *Microscopy Research and Technique, 51*, 101-108.

Smith, C.D. (1996). Quantitative computed tomography and magnetic resonance imaging in aging and Alzheimer's disease: A review. *Journal of Neuroimaging, 6*, 44-53.

Smith, J. (2001). Exercise and atherogenesis. *Exercise & Sport Sciences Reviews, 29*, 49-53.

Smith, M.T., Perlis, M.L., Smith, M.S., Giles, D.E., & Carmody, T.P. (2000). Sleep quality and presleep arousal in chronic pain. *Behavior Medicine, 23(1)*, 1-13.

Soares, J., Holmes, P.V., Renner, K.J., Edwards, G.L., Bunnell, B.N., & Dishman, R.K. (1999). Brain noradrenergic responses to footshock after chronic activity wheel running. *Behavioral Neuroscience, 113*, 558-566

Somberg, B.L., & Salthouse, T.A. (1982). Divided attention abilities in young and old adults. *Journal of Experimental Psychology: Human Perception & Performance, 8*, 651-663.

Sonstroem, R.J. (1997). Physical activity and self-esteem. In W.P. Morgan (Ed.), *Physical activity and mental health* (pp. 127-143). Washington, DC: Taylor & Francis.

Spencer, P.J., Mattsson, J.L., Johnson, K.A., & Albee, R.R. (1993). Neurotoxicity screening methods are sensitive to experimental history. *International Journal of Psychophysiology, 14*, 5-19.

Spirduso, W.W. (1975). Reaction and movement time as a function of age and physical activity level. *Journal of Gerontology, 30 (4)*, 435-440.

Spirduso, W.W. (1980). Physical fitness, aging, and psychomotor speed: A review. *Journal of Gerontology: Medical Sciences, 35(6)*, 850-865.

Spirduso, W.W. (1995). Health, exercise and cognitive functioning. In *Physical dimensions of aging* (pp. 249-273). Champaign, IL: Human Kinetics.

Spirduso, W.W., & Clifford, P. (1978). Replication of age and physical activity effects on reaction and movement time. *Journal of Gerontology: Medical Sciences, 33(1)*, 26-30.

Spirduso, W.W., & Farrar, R.P. (1981). Effects of aerobic training on reactive capacity: An animal model. *Journal of Gerontology, 36*, 654-662.

References

Spirduso, W.W., MacRae, H.H., MacRae, P.G., Prewitt, J., & Osborne, L. (1988). Exercise effects on aged motor function. *Annals of the New York Academy of Sciences, 515,* 363-375.

Spirduso, W.W., Poon, L.W., & Chodzko-Zakjo, W. (Eds.). (in press). *Active living, cognitive functioning, and aging* (Vol. 2). Champaign, IL: Human Kinetics.

Stacey, C., Kozma, A., & Stones, M.J. (1985). Simple cognitive and behavioural changes resulting from improved physical fitness in persons over 50 years of age. *Canadian Journal of Aging, 4,* 67-74.

Sternberg, D.B., Martinez, J.L. Jr., Gold, P.E., & McGaugh, J.L. (1985). Age-related memory deficits in rats and mice: Enhancement with peripheral injections of epinephrine. *Behavioral & Neural Biology, 44,* 213-220.

Stones, M.J., & Kozma, A. (1988). Physical activity, age, and cognitive/motor performance. In M.L. Howe & C.J. Brainerd (Eds.), *Cognitive development in adulthood: Progress in cognitive development research* (pp. 273-321). New York: Springer.

Stones, M.J., & Kozma, A. (1989). Age, exercise and coding performance. *Psychology & Aging, 4,* 190-194.

Strath, S.J., Swartz, A.M., Bassett, D.R. Jr., O'Brien, W.L., King, G.A., & Ainsworth, B.E. (2000). Evaluation of heart rate as a method for assessing moderate intensity physical activity. *Medicine & Science in Sports & Exercise, 32(Suppl. 9),* S465-70S.

Stummer, W., Bauthmann, A., Murr, R., Schurer, L., & Kempski, O.S. (1995). Cerebral protection against ischemia by locomotor activity in gerbils. *Stroke, 26,* 1423-1430.

Sullivan, E.V., Pfefferbaum, A., Adalsteinsson, E., Swan, G.E., & Carmelli, D. (2002). Differential rates of regional change in callosal and ventricular size: A 4-year longitudinal MRI study of elderly men. *Cerebral Cortex, 12,* 438-435.

Surwillo, W.W. (1966). The relation of autonomic activity to age differences in vigilance. *Journal of Gerontology, 21,* 257-260.

Sweeney, J.A., Rosano, C., Berman, R.A., & Luna, B. (2001). Inhibitory control of attention declines more than working memory during normal aging. *Neurobiology of Aging, 22,* 39-47.

Szabo, G., & Hoffmann, P.L. (1995). Brain-derived neurotrophic factor, neurotrophin-3 and neurotrophin-4/5 maintain functional tolerance to ethanol. *European Journal of Pharmacology, 287(1),* 35-41.

Takada, H., Nagata, K., Hirata, Y., Satoh, Y., Watahiki, Y., Sugawara, J., Yokoyama, E., Kondoh, Y., Shishido, F., Inugami, A., Fujita, H., Ogawa, T., Murakami, M., Lida, H., & Kanno, I. (1992). Age-related decline of cerebral oxygen metabolism in normal population detected with positron emission tomography. *Neurological Research, 14,* 128-131.

Tashiro, M., Itoh, M., Fujimoto, T., Fujiwara, T., Ota, H., Kubota, K., Higuchi, M., Okamura, N., Bereczki, D., & Sasaki, H. (2001). 18F-FDG PET mapping of regional brain activity in runners. *Journal of Sports Medicine & Physical Fitness, 41,* 11-17.

References

Taylor, J., Hand, G., Johnson, D., & Seals, D. (1992). Augmented forearm vasoconstriction during dynamic exercise in healthy older men. *Circulation, 86,* 1789-1799.

Tecce, J.J. (1978). Contingent negative variation and attention functions in the aged. In E. Callaway, P. Tueting, & S.H. Koslow (Eds.), *Event-related brain potentials in man.* New York: Academic Press.

Telles, S., Reddy, S.K., & Nagendra, H.R. (2000). Oxygen consumption and respiration following two yoga relaxation techniques. *Applied Psychophysiology & Biofeedback, 25(4),* 221-227.

Thomas, J.R., Landers, D.M., Salazar, W., & Etnier, J. (1994). Exercise and cognitive function. In C. Bouchard, R.J. Shephard, & T. Stephens (Eds.), *Physical activity, fitness, and health: Consensus statement* (pp. 521-529). Champaign, IL: Human Kinetics.

Thornton, J.M., Guz, A., Murphy, K., Giffith, A.R., Pedersen, D.L., Kardos, A., Leff, A., Adams, L., Casadei, B., & Paterson, D.J. (2001). Identification of higher brain centres that may encode the cardiorespiratory response to exercise in humans. *Journal of Physiology, 533,* 823-836.

Tinetti, M.E. (1986). Performance-oriented assessment of mobility problems in elderly patients. *Journal of the American Geriatrics Society, 34,* 119-126.

Tinetti, M.E., Baker, D.I., Gottschalk, M., Williams, C.S., Pollack, D., Garnell, P., Gill, T.M., Marottoli, R.A., & Acampora, D. (1999). Multicomponent rehabilitation program for older persons after hip fracture: A randomized trial. *Archives of Physical Medicine Rehabilitation, 80,* 916-922.

Tinetti, M.E., Speechley, M., & Ginter, S.F. (1988). Risk factors for falls among elderly persons living in the community. *New England Journal of Medicine, 319,* 1701-1707.

Toga, A.W., & Mazziotta, J.C. (Eds.). (2000). *Brain mapping: The systems.* San Diego: Academic Press.

Tomporowski, P.D. (1997). The effects of physical and mental training on the mental abilities of older adults. *Journal of Aging & Physical Activity, 5,* 9-26.

Tomporowski, P.D. (2003). Effects of acute bouts of exercise on cognition. *Acta Psychologica, 112,* 297-324.

Tomporowski, P.D., & Ellis, N.R. (1986). The effects of exercise on cognitive processes: A review. *Psychological Bulletin, 99,* 338-346.

Tong, L., Shen, H., Perreau, V.M., Balazs, R., & Cotman, C.W. (2001). Effects of exercise on gene-expression profile in the rat hippocampus. *Neurobiology of Disease, 8,* 1046-1056.

Tooley, G.A., Armstrong, S.M., Norman, T.R., & Sali, A. (2000). Acute increase in night-time plasma melatonin levels following a period of meditation. *Biological Psychology, 53(1),* 69-78.

Tulving, E., Kapur, S., Craik, F.I.M., Moscovitch, M., & Houle, S. (1994). Hemispheric encoding/retrieval asymmetry in episodic memory: Positron emission tomography findings. *Proceedings of the National Academy of Sciences, 91,* 2016-2020.

Tumer, N., Demirel, H.A., Serova, L., Sabban, E.L., Broxson, C.S., & Powers, S.K. (2001). Gene expression of catecholamine biosynthetic enzymes following exercise: Modulation by age. *Neuroscience, 103,* 703-711.

Upadhyaya, A.K., Conwell, Y., Duberstein, P.R., Denning, D., & Cox, C. (1999). Attempted suicide in older depressed patients: Effect of cognitive functioning. *American Journal of Geriatric Psychiatry, 7(4),* 317-320.

U.S. Department of Health and Human Services. (1996). *Physical activity and health: A report of the surgeon general.* Atlanta: U.S. Department of Health and Human Services, Centers for Disease Control and Prevention, and National Center for Chronic Disease Prevention and Health Promotion.

U.S. Department of Health and Human Services. (2000). *Healthy People 2010: Understanding and improving health* (2nd ed.). Washington, D.C.: Government Printing Office.

Valentino, R.J., & Aston-Jones, G.S. (1995). Physiological and anatomical determinants of locus coeruleus discharge. In F.E. Bloom & D.J. Kupfer (Eds.), *Psychopharmacology: The fourth generation of progress* (pp. 373-385). New York: Raven Press.

van Baar, M.E., Assendelft, W.J., Dekker, J., Oostendorp, R.A., & Bijlsma, J.W. (1999). Effectiveness of exercise therapy in patients with osteoarthritis of the hip or knee: A systematic review of randomized clinical trials. *Arthritis & Rheumatism, 42(7),* 1361-1369.

van Beekvelt, M., Borghuis, M., van Engelen, B., Wevers, R., & Colier, W. (2001). Adipose tissue thickness affects in vivo quantitative near-IR spectroscopy in human skeletal muscle. *Clinical Science (London), 101,* 21-28.

Van Hoomissen, J.D., Holmes, P.V., Zellner, A.S., Poudevigne, A.M., & Dishman, R.K. (2004). Effect of B-adrenergic blockade during chronic exercise on contextual fear conditioning and mRNA for galanin and brain-derived neurotropic factor. *Behavioral Neuroscience, 118,* 1378-1390.

van Praag, H., Christie, B.R., Sejnowski, T.J., & Gage, F.H. (1999). Running enhances neurogenesis, learning, and long-term potentiation in mice. *Proceedings of the National Academy of Sciences, 96,* 13427-13431.

Van Someren, E., Raymann, R., Scherder, E., Daanen, H., & Swaab, D. (2002). Circadian and age-related modulation of thermoreception and temperature regulation: Mechanisms and functional implications. *Ageing Research Reviews, 1(4),* 721-778.

Vempati, R.P., & Telles, S. (2002). Yoga-based guided relaxation reduces sympathetic activity judged from baseline levels. *Psychological Reports, 90(2),* 487-494.

Verbrugge, L.M., & Jette, A.M. (1994). The disablement process. *Social Science & Medicine, 38(1),* 1-14.

Villringer, K., Minoshima, S., Hock, C., Obrig, H., Ziegler, S., Dirnagl, U., Schwaiger, M., & Villringer, A. (1997). Assessment of local brain activation: A simultaneous PET and near infrared spectroscopy study. In A. Villringer & U. Dirnagl (Eds.), *Optical imaging of brain function and metabolism Vol. II* (pp. 149-153). New York: Plenum Press.

References

Vissing, J., Andersen, M., & Diemer, N.H. (1996). Exercise-induced changes in local cerebral glucose utilization in the rat. *Journal of Cerebral Blood Flow & Metabolism, 16,* 729-736.

Vogel, R., Corretti, M., & Plotnik, G. (1997). Effect of a single high-fat meal on endothelial function in healthy subjects. *American Journal of Cardiology, 79,* 350-354.

Vogel, G.W., Neill, D., Hagler, M., Kors, D., & Hartley, D. (1990). Decreased intracranial self-stimulation in a new animal model of endogenous depression. *Neuroscience and Biobehavioral Reviews, 14,* 65-68.

Washburn, R., Chin, M.K., & Montoye, H.J. (1980). Accuracy of pedometers in walking and running. *Research Quarterly for Exercise & Sport, 51,* 695-702.

Washburn, R.A., Goldfield, S.R.W., Smith, K., & McKinlay, J.B. (1990). The validity of exercise induced sweating as a measure of physical activity. *American Journal of Epidemiology, 132,* 107-113.

Washburn, R.A., & Montoye, H.J. (1986). The assessment of physical activity by questionnaire. *American Journal of Epidemiology, 123,* 563-576.

Wasserman, K., Hansen, J., & Sue, J. (1991). Facilitation of oxygen consumption by lactic acidosis during exercise. *News in Physiological Sciences, 6,* 29-34.

Weale, R.A. (1986). Aging and vision. *Vision Research, 26,* 1507-1512.

Weiner, D.K., Bongiomi, D.R., Studenski, S.A., Duncan, P.W., & Kochersberger, G.G. (1993). Does functional reach improve with rehabilitation? *Archives of Physical Medicine Rehabilitation, 74(8),* 796-800.

Weingarten, G. (1973). Mental performance during physical exertion: The benefit of being physically fit. *International Journal of Sport Psychology, 4,* 16-26.

Weiss, J.M., Bonsall, R.W., Demetrikopoulos, M.K., Emery, M.S., & West, C.H.K. (1998). Galanin: A significant role in depression? Annals of the New York Academy of Sciences, *863 (1),* 364-382.

Welk, G.J., Differding, J.A., Thompson, R.W., Blair, S.N., Dziura, J., & Hart, T. (2000). The utility of the Digi-Walker step counter to assess daily physical activity patterns. *Medicine & Science in Sports & Exercise, 32(Suppl.),* S481-S488.

Wenk, G.L. (1989). An hypothesis on the role of glucose in the mechanism of action of cognitive enhancers. *Psychopharmacology, 99,* 431-438.

Werme, M., Thoren, P., Olson, L., & Brene, S. (2000). Running and cocaine both upregulate dynorphin mRNA in medial caudate putamen. *European Journal of Neuroscience, 12,* 2967-2974.

Westerterp, K.R. (1998). Alterations in energy balance with exercise. *American Journal of Clinical Nutrition, 68(4),* 970S-974S.

Westerterp, K.R., Brouns, F., Saris, W.H.M., & Ten Hoor, F. (1988). Comparison of doubly labelled water with respirometry at low- and high-activity levels. *Journal of Applied Physiology, 65,* 53-56.

Westerterp, K.R., de Boer, J.O., Saris, W.H.M., Schoffelen, P.F.M., & Ten Hoor, F. (1984). Measurement of energy expenditure using doubly-labelled water. *International Journal of Sports Medicine, 5(Suppl.),* 74-75.

References

White, A.T., Fehlauer, C.S., Hanover, R.Y., Johnson, S.C., & Dustman, R.E. (1998). Is VO$_2$max an appropriate fitness indicator for older adults? *Journal of Aging and Physical Activity, 6,* 303-309.

White-Welkley, J.E., Warren, G.L., Bunnell, B.N., Mougey, E.H., Meyerhoff, J.L., & Dishman, R.K. (1996). Treadmill exercise training and estradiol increase plasma ACTH and prolactin after novel footshock. *Journal of Applied Physiology, 80,* 931-939.

Wilcox, S., Brenes, G.A., Levine, D., Sevick, M.A., Shumaker, S.A., & Craven, T. (2000). Factors related to sleep disturbance in older adults experiencing knee pain or knee pain with radiographic evidence of knee osteoarthritis. *Journal of the American Geriatrics Society, 48(10),* 1241-1251.

Williamson, J.W., McColl, R., Matthews, D., Mitchell, J.H., Raven, P.B., & Porgan, W.P. (2002). Brain activation by central command during actual and imagined handgrip under hypnosis. *Journal of Applied Physiology, 92,* 1317-1324.

Winder, R., & Borrill, J. (1998). Fuels for memory: The role of oxygen and glucose in memory enhancement. *Psychopharmacology, 136,* 349-356.

Winograd, C.H., Lemsky, C.M., Nevitt, M.C., Nordstrom, T.M., Steward, A.L., Miller, C.J., & Bloch, D.A. (1994). Development of a physical performance and mobility examination. *Journal of the American Geriatrics Society, 42,* 743-749.

Wittig, R.M., Zorick, F.J., Blumer, D., Heilbronn, M., & Roth, T. (1982). Disturbed sleep in patients complaining of chronic pain. *Journal of Nervous & Mental Disorders, 170,* 429-431.

Wolf, E., & Nadroski, A.S. (1971). Extent of the visual field. Changes with age and oxygen tension. *Archives of Ophthalmology, 86,* 637-642.

Woodard, J.L., Grafton, S.T., Votaw, J.R., Green, R.C., Dobraski, M.E., & Hoffman, J.M. (1998). Compensatory recruitment of neural resources during overt rehearsal of word lists in Alzheimer's disease. *Neuropsychology, 12,* 491-504.

World Health Organization. (1997). The Heidelberg guidelines for promoting physical activity among older persons. *Journal of Aging & Physical Activity, 5,* 1, 2-8.

Wright, R.E. (1981). Aging, divided attention, and processing capacity. *Journal of Gerontology, 36,* 605-614.

Yaffe, K., Blackwell, T., Gore, R., Sands, L., Reus, V., & Browner, W.S. (1999). Depressive symptoms and cognitive decline in nondemented elderly women: A prospective study. *Archives of General Psychiatry, 56(5),* 425-430.

Yoo, H.S., Tackett, R.L., Bunnell, B.N., Crabbe, J.B., & Dishman, R.K. (2000). Antidepressant-like effects of physical activity vs. imipramine: Neonatal clomipramine model. *Psychobiology, 28,* 540-549.

Young, A., & Skelton, D.A. (1994). Applied physiology of strength and power in old age. *International Journal of Sports Medicine, 15(3),* 149-151.

Zakzanis, K.K., Graham, S.J., & Campbell, Z. (2003). A meta-analysis of structural and functional brain imaging in dementia of the Alzheimer's type: A neuroimaging profile. *Neuropsychology Review, 13,* 1-18.

Ziegler, M., Lake, C., & Kopin, I. (1976). Plasma norepinephron increases with age. *Nature, 261,* 333-335.

INDEX

Italicized *f* and *t* refer to figure and table, respectively.

Leonard W. Poon, PhD, is professor of psychology, director of the Gerontology Center, and chair of the faculty of gerontology at the University of Georgia. A fellow of the American Psychological Association, American Psychological Society, Association of Gerontology in Higher Education, and the Gerontology Society of America, Dr. Poon was a Fulbright senior research scholar in Sweden and a senior visiting research scientist to Japan. Among his research awards are the NIA Special Research Award, VA Medical Research Service Achievement Award, North American Leader in Psychogeriatrics, 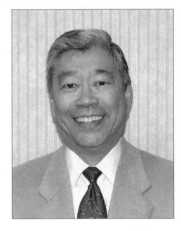 and Southern Gerontological Society Academic Gerontologist Award. His primary research areas are in normal and pathological changes of memory processes in aging, clinical assessment of memory (including assessment of early stages of dementia of the Alzheimer's type), and survival characteristics and adaptation of centenarians. He is currently directing a nine-university, NIA-funded program studying the genetic basis of longevity, relationships between the brain and behavior in Alzheimer's disease, and daily functioning capacities of the oldest old.

Wojtek Chodzko-Zajko, PhD, serves as both department head and professor of kinesiology and community health at the University of Illinois at Urbana-Champaign. He served on the World Health Organization Scientific Advisory Committee, which issued guidelines for physical activity in older adults. He chairs the Active Aging Partnership, a national coalition in the area of healthy aging linking the American College of Sports Medicine, the National Institute of Aging, the Centers for Disease Control and Prevention, the American Geriatrics Society, the National Council on the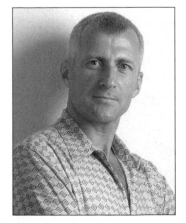

Aging, the American Association of Retired Persons, and the Robert Wood Johnson Foundation

Since 2002, Dr. Chodzko-Zajko has served as principal investigator of the National Blueprint Project, a coalition of more than 50 national organizations with a joint commitment to promoting independent, active aging in the 50+ population. He was founding editor of the *Journal of Aging and Physical Activity* and president of the International Society for Aging and Physical Activity.

He is frequently invited to speak about healthful aging at national and international meetings. Dr. Chodzko-Zajko also has appeared often on television and radio, including the NBC "Today Show," National Public Radio, and CNN.

Phillip D. Tomporowski, PhD, associate professor at the University of Georgia, specializes in the study of the effects of physical activity on mental functioning in children, individuals diagnosed as mentally retarded, and older adults. He served on the editorial board of the *Journal of Aging and Physical Activity*.

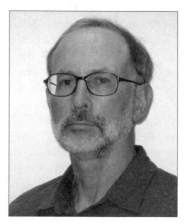

Dr. Tomporowski is the author of *Psychology of Skill: A Life-Span Approach* (2003). His many publications include a review of papers describing the relation between exercise and cognitive functioning and empirical research addressing the relation between physical activity and aging.